Multiple Sclerosis
Through History and Human Life

May 20, 1919

My legs have to be tied to the bed
with a rope. A little girl staying here
lends me her skipping rope.

W. N. P. Barbellion,
The Journal of a Disappointed Man

Multiple Sclerosis Through History and Human Life

by RICHARD M. SWIDERSKI

McFarland & Company, Inc., Publishers
Jefferson, North Carolina, and London

Acknowledgments: This book grew out of, and beyond, my discovery that I was linked with many other people in having MS. My knowledge of this state of being is constantly questioned and advanced by links with other MS people through on-line correspondence and conversations in small rooms. My thanks go to Janet, Ellen, Michael, Terry, Joyce, Giselle and Dieter for the chance to hold hands and to Joolie for facilitating many of the contacts. After the book was written I profited from the chance to talk with Tina, Margie, Donald, Richard, Lorna, Janelle and David.

In the world of paper, Claire Nutt of Wellcome Institute in London provided a seed bibliography, and Robin Chandler of the University of California–San Francisco gave me access to several antique volumes that opened up the early years of the disease.

I would like to express special gratitude to Dorothy ("Muz") Olayos, who spoke with me about her son Vernon and gave me a copy of the book she made from his diary. I dedicate this book to Vernon's memory.

British Library Cataloguing-in-Publication data are available

Library of Congress Cataloguing-in-Publication Data

Swiderski, Richard M.
    Multiple sclerosis through history and human life / by Richard M. Swiderski.
        p.   cm.
    Includes bibliographical references and index.
    ISBN 0-7864-0562-7 (sewn softcover : 50# alkaline paper) ∞
    1. Multiple sclerosis — History.   2. Multiple sclerosis — Patients.
I. Title.
RA645.M82S95   1998
616.8'34'009 — dc21   98-37977
                                                                    CIP

Manufactured in the United States of America

McFarland & Company, Inc., Publishers
    Box 611, Jefferson, North Carolina 28640

Contents

Introduction:
The World of
Multiple Sclerosis

There is always the possibility that a cure will be invented and that multiple sclerosis (MS) will join smallpox, leprosy and (we hope) polio as a disease of the past. But other diseases once thought to be "of the past" include tuberculosis and syphilis.

At present, a cure for multiple sclerosis is difficult to imagine. It would require detecting and halting damage to nerve tissue and restoring the tissue that has been damaged — as well as restoring the withered muscles, blind eyes and wracked bladders of those who have been trapped by the disease, not to mention restoring the shattered marriages, reuniting the alienated families, rebuilding the broken careers, recovering the forgotten skills and paying back the money spent but never earned. Most people with MS, however, would be pleased just to have their nerves working again, to be able to see clearly and walk unaided — and not to be depressed.

Because of these anguishes, MS is a well-known disease in those parts of the world where it occurs. Because those parts of the world are affluent and technologically sophisticated, multiple sclerosis is a well-known disease indeed. It is a toss-up whether the widespread knowledge of MS in these areas is due to its great frequency or to the success of the MS societies in disseminating information. The prevalence is given as 50–90 cases per 10,000 people in Great Britain and the United States (Kesselring 1997:1, also expressed as 1 case per 800).

In the American milieu it seems that actual prevalence of the disease and information about it are interrelated. The National Multiple Sclerosis Society, headquartered in New York with hundreds of regional societies and local chapters spread throughout the country, keeps public attention focused on the

1

plight of those with multiple sclerosis while providing support and encouragement through discussion groups and legal aid. Today, people diagnosed with MS seem less hesitant and more able to identify themselves than they were during the decades before the founding of the society in 1946.

When I tell someone in the United States that I have MS, that person is likely to know, or know of, someone else also living with the disease. This is a sad commentary on its frequency but a happy commentary on the freedom to mention the disease openly. At least those others with MS are known to be living.

This attitude toward MS has found a representation in American celebrity culture. When Annette Funicello, famous to the post–World War II baby-boom generation as an early television star (*The Mickey Mouse Club*), announced she had received an MS diagnosis, she simultaneously updated her celebrity status and became an effective fund-raiser for the Multiple Sclerosis Society. Her autobiography, *A Dream Is a Wish Your Heart Makes* (1994), quoted an old Disney movie song in its title, to merge one American genre, the celebrity life history (about the American dream), with another, younger genre, the personal multiple sclerosis story.

If celebrities can have multiple sclerosis, anyone can. The caustic comic Richard Pryor admitted to his multiple sclerosis in the wake of a near-fatal burn and played a multiple sclerosis patient in an episode of a television hospital series. The singers Donna Fargo and Lola Falana, the politician Barbara Jordan, the cyclist Mo Manly and the skier Jimmy Heuga were among the more specialized celebrities who became publicly associated with the condition, helping to create an atmosphere in which having multiple sclerosis is not so strange and not an insuperable affliction.

Being interested in the arts, I could recall that the cellist Jacqueline duPre ended her career due to multiple sclerosis and that the novelist and essayist Stanley Elkin not only had the disease but incorporated his experience into his writings. Nancy Mairs' literary essays and autobiography place her own multiple sclerosis in the context of a woman's and a disabled person's self-discovery. Being occupied with public events, I could notice that Joe Hartzler, the U.S. Department of Justice attorney and chief prosecutor in the trial of the men accused of bombing a federal building in Oklahoma City, is also laboring under the burden of multiple sclerosis. I could note the names of a number of businesspeople, stockbrokers and real estate agents, well-known within their spheres, who have the disease. The investigative journalist Ellen Burstein MacFarlane, having taken false hope from a doctor, turned her experience into an exposé. And continuing with the news, Dr. Jack Kevorkian counts a number of MS sufferers among the people he has "helped to die." All aspects of the multiple sclerosis experience and its effects on various Americans are visible in the newspapers, magazines and books, on television and even occasionally in the movies.

The U.S. multiple sclerosis sphere encloses a continuing drama of life with multiple sclerosis, including the search for an effective treatment. When the writer Dian Smith (1995) came to terms with her mother's death from multiple sclerosis, she telephoned a medical research unit to ask if it needed donations of multiple sclerosis tissue to forward work on a cure. That cure is the aim most alive in the minds of those who fund, pursue and monitor multiple sclerosis research, just as it is for those in cancer or AIDS research, in varying degrees of investment strategy and personal urgency.

Because multiple sclerosis destroys some of its victims with uncertain slowness, these victims are awake to watch efforts being made on their behalf and are eager to participate in these efforts, especially if participation might yield relief. At public libraries and on the Internet, indices list research studies on multiple sclerosis and on many other chronic diseases and give the names and addresses of the researchers so that potential volunteers can contact them. Unlike the drug-addiction treatment studies, which must advertise for paid volunteers in major urban newspapers, multiple sclerosis research seems to have an ample cadre of volunteers just among patients at multiple sclerosis and neurology clinics.

Researchers never claim to plan a cure, just to try to reduce damage or bring relief from symptoms. Their most publicized efforts, and those that attract the most funding, concentrate on drugs. It has long been known that physical exercise and diet control have positive effects on all but the most advanced cases of MS, and the MS societies as well as most doctors and nurses spread this information. But this knowledge always takes a backseat to the hope for a pill that will wipe away the effects of the disease. Side effects and cost are far less important than the hope that multiple sclerosis can be banished with ease and simplicity through directed consumption of a prepared commercial package.

When the Berlex Company (a division of Hoffmann–La Roche) announced in 1992 that it would begin distributing betaseron, a synthetic interferon beta newly approved for multiple sclerosis treatment, the response from patients and therapists was so insistent that the company had to set up a lottery. Names filed with authorized physicians were put into a nationwide bin and drawn at random to decide who would receive doses of the drug. The usual questions arose. Would insurance companies and health maintenance organizations pay for the treatments? How much would they cover? There were stories of both greed and selflessness as some people plotted to secure doses for themselves while others ceded their betaseron to people more in need.

Berlex set up an 800 telephone line with a menu of recorded announcements explaining the lottery and offering detailed information on all aspects of the drug. Local multiple sclerosis societies added betaseron support groups to their monthly schedules.

After a year of lottery-driven dosage, the news was disappointing.

Betaseron was not as effective in alleviating fatigue and loss of coordination as its tests suggested, and its side effects raised some qualms. Betaseron joined many other medications used at doctors' discretion in treating particular cases. Treatment knowledge of the drug entered physicians' common practice, enabling them to understand better whom it would benefit and whom it might harm. The concurrent availability of the powerful antidepressants Prozac and Zoloft added a chance to escape depression for some. Soon betaseron was joined by Avonex and copolymer, which had their own styles of administration and their own success claims.

The betaseron episode was widely publicized in newspapers. Its elements of chance, eager consumption and the possible triumph of a new technology over a well-known disease describe the American world of MS. Scientific knowledge, mediated by newspapers and nonprofit associations, is devoured in processed form by a large number of people suffering personally or socially from a disease that they know national resources must someday defeat. For now, they struggle to live and work despite a disease rooted in common human biology. We have always been able to work biology as we want to. It just takes time. This summarizes the present approach to multiple sclerosis, at least in America.

The epigraph of the International Forum of Multiple Sclerosis Societies (IFMSS) reads, "Multiple sclerosis is the same disease everywhere." That is a fundamental tenet of the scientific view of multiple sclerosis maintained in North America and Europe. The 43 member societies of the International Forum certainly believe that the multiple sclerosis they address is the same everywhere: the Japan Multiple Sclerosis Society is aiding people afflicted by exactly the same disease that is afflicting those helped by the Torkiye Multipl Skleroz Dernegi of Turkey or the Multiple Sclerosis Felag Islands of Iceland. That the French have their Ligue Française Contre la Sclérose en Plaques and the Poles have their Polskie Towarzystwo Stwardienia Roszaniego is a difference only in names and not in condition addressed. The societies expanded from the first ones founded in the United States (1946) and Great Britain (1953) with the purpose of informing the public about multiple sclerosis, helping multiple sclerosis patients and influencing government action in favor of those disabled by multiple sclerosis. The national societies in Mexico, Japan and now eastern Europe often were motivated by U.S. or British expatriates: the multiple sclerosis *Update* of the IFMSS reported a St. Petersburg society founded with the help of a British physician. The pamphlets distributed by the Mexican society are Spanish translations of U.S. English pamphlets. In responding to my request for information, the secretary of the Japan Multiple Sclerosis Society stated quite plainly that the Japanese learned about multiple sclerosis from foreigners.

The disease is the same demyelination everywhere (allowing for name-pathology mismatches caused by misdiagnosis), but the sickness and the illness aren't the same everywhere. *Sickness* is the word that medical social scientists use to designate the social construction of the biological disease. The distinction allows for culturally different responses to disease while avoiding claims of radical culturalism (that the representation is the only reality of disease). *Illness* is the individual course of the disease, obviously under the spell of both personal biology and cultural difference at the same time.

The Japanese may suffer from demyelination, but the expression of the resultant pain is a Japanese expression and the social treatment of the sufferer is within Japanese institutions. The rarity of multiple sclerosis in Japan compared with the United States or Britain also affects its course as a sickness. Information about the disease is not as widespread as in countries with a higher prevalence. A person is diagnosed with multiple sclerosis by a doctor and then, together with the family, learns about it and receives assistance from the multiple sclerosis society. This alone contributes to making MS a different sickness in Japan. From Japanese publications it is possible to learn how the groups — but not the individuals — feel about MS.

Throughout this book, multiple sclerosis as sickness and illness will be balanced against multiple sclerosis as disease. The three have been quite intricately confounded in the United States and Great Britain, where it is assumed that multiple sclerosis, being the same disease everywhere, is also the same sickness everywhere and is the same illness that our celebrities (or friends with MS) suffer.

Although the causes of and potential cures for the disease are resolutely pursued in many places (the Turkish national multiple sclerosis society funds the work of young multiple sclerosis researchers), the manner of that pursuit and the context of the biological disease vary greatly. As many times as the uniformity of the disease is asserted, the variety of the sickness and illness seems to transform it into many different diseases. The cliché that multiple sclerosis is idiosyncratic and affects each person differently overlies an assumption that it has a single cause.

The same might be said of the national multiple sclerosis societies. Some — the Japanese and the Indian societies — are the sole outposts of multiple sclerosis where it is quite uncommon. The Indian society more or less confines its attentions to the Parsee community, which has a much higher rate of affliction than the general population of India. The only sub–Saharan African multiple sclerosis societies are in South Africa and Zambia, where they serve concentrations of people of European ancestry. Other societies, such as those of Britain or Sweden, represent repositories of information and aid for the common sufferer. Multiple sclerosis affects each nation differently, and yet it is the same underlying disease. During his heyday as a diagnostician, Jean-Martin Charcot received multiple sclerosis patients from China, yet today China has no national multiple sclerosis society, nor does Iran or Russia, where there is some amount of multiple sclerosis.

The Ligue Française Contre la Sclérose en Plaques was founded only in 1986, decades after the English and American societies; with an estimated total multiple sclerosis population of 50,000, it has only 575 members. Controlled by male academics and doctors, it is a small, elite organization, which arranges services and assistance for most of the people afflicted with the disease, in a way continuing the clinical approach established by Charcot during the late nineteenth century. The lateness of the French society also suggests something about the evolution of relations between physicians, patients and public authority in France.

The Deutsche Multiple Sklerose Gesellschaft was founded at about the same time (1952) as the British and American societies; it has over 35,000 members from a total estimated multiple sclerosis population of 120,000. Academic doctors figure prominently in the association, and some of them are women. The services extended are similar to those of other associations: help and advice. In addition to the multiple sclerosis centers, this society offers health resorts, an established tradition for chronic disease treatment in Germany and in the Scandinavian countries. The German society, like the British and American societies, supports many local multiple sclerosis associations. This is a function not only of the large German general population (several times that of France or Britain): Germans with multiple sclerosis are more likely to join their association than are the French. In the Scandinavian and Polish societies, which are dedicated to neurological disease in general, the membership of the societies exceeds the multiple sclerosis population by several times. Family, friends and other supporters join the societies to take part in their events. This too reflects long-standing traditions of coping with chronic illness in these societies.

The bare statistics of the national multiple sclerosis societies alone give a profile of the differences in multiple sclerosis as a sickness throughout the world. The narrow diagnostic history of the disease intersects with the even more complex social and cultural history of the sickness — how it is like other sicknesses and how it is unique.

The disease itself has a history that interacts with these social and individual dimensions. The disease is not the same everywhere. It is affected by different genetics, environment and diet; by different development in the child and the adult; and by different diagnostic standards. There is a world of multiple sclerosis, but it is not clearly centered around a single absolute disease entity from which everyone who has multiple sclerosis suffers.

Multiple sclerosis has both a long and a short history: the history within anyone's lifetime, and the cumulative history since it was first noticed. The short history known to a sufferer or an interested other contains many elements of the long one. I cannot hope to compose a complete history of MS, but I do wish to look beyond the short history that many of us develop, to see what other multiple scleroses there have been and are. I do this with the understanding that there is always healing in knowledge and always knowledge in the attempt to heal.

What I hope this book accomplishes is consistent with the aims of the more humane multiple sclerosis societies: to abolish the disease while hearing what those who live with it have to say. The whole history is not just a movement toward the present-day pinnacle of knowledge. It is made up of many worlds of disease, illness and sickness. This history, drawn from the copious records of sufferers, companions, healers and other historians, can only begin to show those worlds.

1

The Earliest MS

In 1947, during the civic reconstruction that followed World War II, there was discovered in the Dutch town of Schiedam (now a suburb of Rotterdam) a woman's skeleton showing distinct abnormalities. It was not until 1957 that the skeleton was analyzed anatomically at the University of Leiden. Signs of severe loss of muscle mass and related bone distortion pointed to paralysis of both legs. Comparable signs in the arm and shoulder suggested that the right side may have been paralyzed as well (DeWilde 1958).

The skeleton was identified as that of Lidwina van Schiedam, a "pious virgin" known to have lived from 1380 to 1433. In a local charter dated August 4, 1421, "Jan van Beieren, Count of Holland, confirms a letter of the local authorities of Schiedam which dealt with 'the strange disease of the virgin Lidwina'" (Medaer 1979:189). Examining van Beieren's account and a biography of the saint by the Franciscan Johannes Brugman, together with the skeletal evidence, the Flemish neurologist R. Medaer concluded that Lidwina suffered from multiple sclerosis.

On February 2, 1395, Lidwina, then 15 years old, fell while ice skating and broke one of her ribs. The abscess that formed at the place of the fracture healed only slowly and with great difficulty. Lidwina had trouble walking and suffered lacerating tooth pains. The best physicians could not heal her. By the time she was 19, her difficulties in walking had worsened, and she had a "split face" and a "hanging lip," which Medaer interprets as indicative of facial paralysis. Her right eye went blind, and her left was oversensitive to light. Soon she had to be carried wherever she went.

After 1407 Lidwina exhibited the ability to be in two places at once, to levitate over her bed and to have conversations with God and angels. During and after these "exstases," Lidwina's eyesight and movement improved. These events seem to have fixed in the minds of her family and community that Lidwina's illness came directly from God. The Franciscan chronicler Brugman, whose information came secondhand from Lidwina's confessor and from various neighbors and relatives, was making a case for Lidwina's sainthood, which would require a minimum number of documented proofs of divine election.

In the year 1413 large wounds appeared on Lidwina's body; these, together with swallowing difficulties and other pains, continued until the end of her life. Medaer sensibly offers the interpretation of decubitus or bedsores for the wounds. The description of the other pains, he believes, is consistent with renal blockage, and hard swallowing is typical of people in the later stages of MS.

For Medaer, "the described symptoms cannot find an explanation in other diseases than multiple sclerosis. Paralysis of both legs, paralysis of the right arm, facial paralysis, blindness with different gradations in both eyes, sensibility disturbances, difficulties in swallowing may very well be explained by various affections in the white matter of the central nervous system."

Physical trauma often precipitates an awareness of MS. The apparent beginning of Lidwina's affliction was her skating accident. She was a healthy and charming young girl before that accident. That she was rather young for the onset of MS does not deter Medaer: at 15 years of age, she fell within the MS age range of between 10 and 50. Though Medaer does not mention it, the fact that Lidwina was a woman and a Northerner by birth would also add credibility to the diagnosis. If MS existed that long ago, then it can't be a newly developing disease.

That Lidwina's case was preceded by an abscess is curious. The clinical neurology manual that Medaer consulted (Schumacher in Baker 1962) follows Charcot in finding a physical trauma at the root of MS, leading to the other symptoms that Medaer lists. Studies of MS cases (Jellinek 1994) have revealed, however, that few actually were precipitated by a trauma: that event may only bring the presence of the symptoms dramatically to notice. A blow or a sprain will trigger a slight seizure, a ringing in the ears and sweating as well as shock symptoms in people with nerve damage. Many nerve disorders besides MS can induce symptoms like Lidwina's.

The abscess with attendant bacterial infection at the beginning of Lidwina's travails introduces an alternative explanation: systemic infection. Another writer, the Reverend Alban Butler, examining the same sources as Medaer but with a devotional intent, describes the complications of her skating accident as follows: "From which hurt, accompanied by an inward bruise and from a great impostume formed in the womb, she suffered extremely, taking very little nourishment and struggling day and night" (Butler 1904: vol. 4, 88). The impostume or tumor in the womb might have been enough to put pressure on nerves to the leg, causing paralysis. Since there was no method of containing infections during that period, a lingering staphylococcus center might have affected her limb muscles, leading to disuse and the bone attenuation observed in her remains, and might have caused further infections in her eyes, teeth and throat as well as the rash of sores, which at least could be held in check through external treatment. The failure to take food for long periods would have increasingly severe health consequences, which, short of death, might lead to remarkable states of mind and body. Medaer focuses so closely on having the first documented case of MS that he does not even consider the alternatives.

There is also a question about the chronology of Lidwina's symptoms. The official sources give a rough chronological sequence, but the ecclesiastical accounts adhere to hagiographic tradition and present their somewhat richer detail grouped according to allegorical classes: her body was cloven in three to represent schism in the Catholic Church; and each section of the body suffered in accordance with the institution it represented.

Saints besides Lidwina were afflicted with bizarre physical symptoms and experienced attendant ecstasies. Such a combination of effects in that time could be either divine or demonic in origin. The Franciscan hagiographer Brugman cites Sonderdank, the Burgundian court physician who attended Lidwina, as stating that it was impossible to heal the woman through human efforts, that God had touched her.

In 1417 the last Count of Holland died, leaving a power vacuum that the Burgundians filled for a time, hence the role of Sonderdank examining the center of a local Dutch cult. The Franciscan biographer is making his politically appropriate case for the sainthood of the woman, long deceased by the time his biography went through the first of its three editions. Lidwina was a virgin vessel chosen to suffer torments for all and to enjoy the foretaste of heaven in her ecstasies. This was one of the few ways a woman might gain this experience: directly through the body. Without a declaration of God's hand, it could only be the devil's work.

Lidwina died a holy virgin at the age of 52 (four days short of her 53rd birthday). According to Brugman, she had already declared at age 12, her wish to be a virgin. She would have been a burden to her father unless her sanctity could be promoted well enough to attract donations and pilgrims. Developing a cult would also be a boon to Schiedam, which lacked a holy figure of its own before Lidwina's appearance. Driven by its success as a port in the grain and fish trade, Schiedam was organizing its municipal religion. Schiedam's main place of worship, the Groote Kerk (Sant Janskerk), was consecrated in 1400. There was every reason to cultivate Lidwina's remarkable condition and spread abroad rumors of her sanctity, insights and miracles while she was alive and to codify her legend in the conventions of sainthood after her death.

Those conventions had long been developed by the medieval church to identify the lives of people chosen by God. The church itself did not claim the ability to work miracles and was thus open to individuals with interesting lives adaptable to saintly manifestations. For every Lidwina who succeeded in the prophetic career, there must have been hundreds of others who genuinely suffered from a range of afflictions or who attempted to convince others that they were inspired but whom we have never heard of enough to match their lives with their preserved remains and arrive at a modern diagnosis.

Lidwina's reputation persisted long enough for the Dutch monk Thomas à Kempis to write his *Vita Lidewigis Virginis* (1448) 15 years after her death. Best known as the "probable" author of *Imitatio Christi*, the most widely read Christian book after the Bible, Thomas was born in the year of Lidwina's accident (1380) and lived most of his long life (d. 1473) in the Augustinian monastery near Zwolle, on the Ijssel River some distance to the northwest of Schiedam. It is conceivable that Thomas visited Lidwina — his *Vita* gives eye-witness accounts of several miracles — though his book clearly is based on Brugman's biography. As a member of the contemplative and antimaterialist Brethren of the Common Life, and a teacher of direct emulation of the model of Christ in everyday life, Thomas would not have approved of Lidwina's mystical ecstasies.

She was fortunate or skilled to avoid the fate of other women who exhibited such behavior and were executed as witches during this most intense era of the European witch craze. It may well be that witchcraft and demonic possession covered MS and a great variety of other behaviors some of us today ascribe to neurological disorders. Witchcraft and possession were a way for the body politic to explain and act on individual deviations from the perceived norm. These supernatural ascriptions had their own logic and diagnostics, which seem primitive because they were not careful of the physical realities.

Despite the support of Brugman, Thomas and others, Lidwina was not canonized a saint until 1895 (the German mystic Hildegard von Bingen never was). She remained a Holy Virgin (feast day April 14) listed in the more detailed church calendars, and her bones retained their identification for centuries, surviving Protestantism's rout of superstitious relics. In the vast list of saints, she became the patron saint of ice skaters.

The case of the virgin Lidwina shows Medaer's determination to project the clinical-anatomical method of diagnosis backward in time in the search for early MS cases, which means that MS was included with the many other diseases being sought in the same way. But the problem with this approach, even with some anatomical data at hand, is discerning the physical disease in the cultural sickness and assuming we know the disease then. Lidwina's contemporaries were busy converting sickness into hagiography, just as Medaer was busy converting hagiography into medical case history.

Did Lidwina really have MS? There is no way to tell for sure. The answer hinges on accepting her bone deformations as paralysis, her paralysis as neural in nature, her vision loss as optic neuritis, her ecstasies as the equivalent of MS euphoria and sensory excitements and the remitting-relapsing course of her sickness as an MS cycle and not as a chronic infection or a metabolic-nutritional condition of a completely different sort.

In favor of Medaer's interpretation, however, I would only add that during their first MS exacerbations, people can feel as if their bodies are being commanded by an outside force. I know one MS-afflicted woman who was sure she was possessed by a demon who drew the energy out of her legs and the insides of her eyes before a nurse convinced her it was a condition of her nerves. Those of a religious bent seem to choose the devil more often than God to explain the bodily state of incipient MS. A reading of the personal histories of MS victims confirms this. Just as sanctity and then sainthood absorbed Lidwina's life, religious beliefs may have subsumed many another person's understanding of the causes of a bodily state.

Something of the transition from Catholic hagiography to medical case record can be felt in the novel that Joris Karl Huysmans, the French novelist of Dutch descent (born of a French mother and Dutch father in Paris, he wrote in French), wrote about Lidwina. Huysmans was one of the chief figures in the fin-de-siècle Symbolist movement in France. At first under the influence of the poet Baudelaire, he was attracted to the naturalism of Emile Zola and wrote novels that combined the two influences. His best-known work is fiction and art criticism consumed with decadence, the weary indulgence of all the senses. He published *Sainte Lydwine van Schiedam* in 1901, after an agonized reconversion to Catholicism and entry into a religious brotherhood.

Against an apocalyptic fin de siècle (fourteenth or nineteenth century) backdrop, Huysmans describes the extremes of Lidwina's physical and spiritual anguish, setting them off against her mystical ecstasies. He translates the sensual extremes of literary hyperesthesia into Catholic hagiography. The paintings of Matthias Grünewald, especially his *Temptation of Saint Anthony*, which Huysmans wrote about before his conversion, seem to provide Huysmans with his vision of Lidwina. In taking up Lidwina, Huysmans is also returning to the Dutch ethnic identity he flirted with all his life.

Medaer's MS diagnosis of Lidwina is a medicalization of her life history paralleling Huysmans' translation of that same life into naturalist language, which approaches clinical language. Medaer, a Fleming in Belgium, appears to be claiming the first identifiable case of MS as Dutch. The importance of the national identity of MS and of its diagnosticians will recur with growing insistence throughout this history. It is one more way for the cultural to be made biological while remaining cultural.

The clinical-anatomical inspection of a past life is one obvious way to study MS prehistory. It may move the past into more concretely immediate experience, at the risk of ignoring some important details about the past, which also may be ignored in the present. Medaer saw only the MS he knew in Lidwina. Another way to seek MS before anyone knew what it was is to link past events with present-day patterns.

The epidemiology of MS, better defined all the time, exhibits some suggestive patterns. Best known is the tendency of the disease to favor the northern latitudes and to be more likely to develop in people who were born and lived in these regions and then migrated south. The epidemiology can be interpreted in terms of a documented historical pattern of migration to suggest genetic or other transmission, much as the peculiarities of an exhumed skeleton can be interpreted in terms of a recorded biography to give a trace of a past disease.

Charles Poser, a neuroepidemiologist at Harvard University Medical School, in several articles (Poser 1994; Poser 1995; Shakir, Newman and Poser 1996) has argued that a genetically mediated susceptibility to MS is a more consistent explanation of the worldwide distribution of the disease than distribution by latitude. The universal of environment is therefore replaced by the variable of history. For Poser, the historical distribution is not arbitrary. Noting the greater frequency of MS in populations of Scandinavian descent, he postulates that the most widely traveled Scandinavians and those most likely to spread their genes into other populations, the Vikings, determined the pattern of MS susceptibility throughout the world.

Poser does not claim that the Vikings carried a single MS gene or even that they themselves had cases of MS. Through their widespread raids into northern Europe and as far south as Sicily and northern Africa, their slave-taking and -trading and their military activities in what became Russia, Byzantium and the Mongol Empire, the Vikings "may have contributed to the dissemination of MS throughout the world" (Poser 1995:21).

Poser cites only one instance of a woman's temporary blindness, described in the Icelandic saga of St. Thorlakr (Poser 1995:12). This is his only sally into vague textual evidence interpretable as MS, in the manner of Medaer. Most of his data are historical studies of the spread of the Vikings during their period of expansion from the eighth to the tenth century A.D. and the correlation of these advances and incursions with some regularities and peculiarities of MS epidemiology.

Poser's articles are devoted to demonstrating, through presentation of the historical sources, how Viking genetic material could have found its way far enough and wide enough to influence contemporary MS rates. This evidence establishes a Viking touch where MS also can be documented. Varangian runes on a marble lion in the Venetian Piraeus and a runic inscription on a marble screen in Hagia Sophia, Istanbul, show that Vikings were in the Mediterranean. Proof that the Canary Islands were settled by Normans correlates well with the higher-than-expected prevalence of MS there.

Drawing on his own research in Kuwait (Al Din, Kogali and Poser 1991), Poser postulates that the rate of MS among Palestinian Arabs living in Kuwait, nearly two and a half times that of Kuwaiti Arabs, is explained by the Palestinians' origins in the Crusaders' (Normans, originally Vikings) Latin kingdom of Jerusalem. The Palestinians' tendency to have lighter-colored eyes than neighboring Arabs supports the presence of other hereditary influences.

This difference in MS rates occurs despite the fact that Kuwaiti Arabs and Kuwaiti Palestinians were raised in the same environment. A genetically mediated susceptibility to MS is Poser's preferred explanation of these data.

A Viking dissemination of hereditarily transmissible susceptibility to MS would also help account for the varying rates in Great Britain and the United States. There is a south-to-north increasing gradient of prevalence in England, which corresponds with the intensity of Viking invasion and conquest. The pre–Columbian Viking incursions on the eastern coast of America did not lead to any long-lasting settlements. Native Americans have the lowest MS rate of any known group. The eventual migration of Scandinavians into the United States and their concentrated settlement in the midwestern states may have led to a relatively elevated rate in those areas.

More data can match contemporary rates with past migrations, but by Poser's own admission, the correlation is general rather than precise. There is no one hereditary material that can be traced from Viking ancestors to MS cases today, but a quest for any such substance would be best pursued along these lines. Poser's genetic postulate is the other major way to compose a biocultural history of MS. Instead of setting up the informational requirements characteristic of the anatomical-clinical method (anatomical remains and written accounts of cases), he imagines a substance or set of substances spread and infiltrated into populations through historic movements and settlement practices of a specific group. Assuming that this substance is genetic puts aside any question of its origins and makes it possible for its precise nature to remain speculatively vague. By seeking a biochemical common ground among all those afflicted with MS today and their Viking forebears, the genetic hypothesis gives MS an ancient history.

It is very difficult to try to verify Poser's hypothesis by performing biochemical assays of long deceased people. It does leave the possibility that some traceable chemistry can be detected, as it once was possible to imagine traceable MS anatomical peculiarities. To provide a prehistory of MS and a credible genetics, Poser must maintain the vagueness of the substance and postulate interactions with other genetics, environmental factors and other illnesses to generate MS as we know it.

The earliest MS must be an extension backward of what we know of MS today, primarily because the characteristics of the disease were defined only recently and thus any scanning of the past must be a backward projection of present knowledge. These methods are very revealing about the nature of this search even in the present. Biology is always defined culturally, in terms of a symptomatology or a hypothesized transmissible protein set. But culture, in turn, is defined biologically: the symptoms are the special property of a group; the genes are activated by voyages and mating patterns. An understanding of early MS, as long as it remains speculative, reflects the intricate intermingling of culture and biology.

Iceland is one of the few nation-states remaining on the planet: that is, its population and citizens are all members of the same ethnic group. Since it was settled by Vikings in 874 A.D. and since then has been rather isolated the inbred Icelanders could serve as a test of Poser's hypothesis. The incidence of MS is comparatively high, but do sufferers share a unique gene? An Icelandic physician, Kari Stefansson, formerly a professor at Harvard medical school, has formed a biotechnology company, Decode Genetics, to study the DNA of Icelanders in search of genetic clues to MS, diabetes and other diseases (*Wall Street Journal*, July 10, 1996: B1;B9). The population is small enough and historically well enough tracked to permit tracing gene lines back to Viking founders. But the aim of the company is not historical research; it's seeking those portions of the genome which could be targeted by drugs. The ancient history of MS in Iceland is only meaningful if it leads to a treatment.

2

MS Comes to Notice

In 1818 the professor of anatomy and physiology at Glasgow University, James Jeffray, performed what was to be the last public dissection of an executed murderer. Jeffray was a popular lecturer who knew how to dramatize his displays and on this occasion he demonstrated "animal electricity" by administering to the corpse a jolt of electricity from a voltaic pile. The corpse abruptly sat upright, and with the audience in a frenzy, Jeffray cut the corpse's neck, causing it to collapse. Perhaps the impression left by this or similar galvanic demonstrations was stirred again by the publication of Mary Shelley's *Frankenstein; or, The New Prometheus* in that same year ("I saw the yellow eye of the creature open; it breathed hard, and a convulsive motion agitated its limbs").

Luigi Galvani had interpreted his discovery (1791) that frog legs jerk when in contact with two different metals as a sign of the existence of electricity within the animal muscle, and Alessandro Volta had in turn proven (1794) that the two metals could generate a current without the animal tissue. Jeffray wasn't performing an experiment with the corpse; he was just putting on a show, as "electricians" had long done. Curiously, however, Emil Du Bois-Reymond, the researcher who was to discover the electrical nature of nerve impulses and initiate another phase of MS history, was born in 1818.

Jeffray liked to have a record of his accomplishments. Robert Carswell, a young Paisley man, showed such skill making drawings of Jeffray's (abortive) boat-propelling device and then of anatomical models that Jeffray encouraged him to enter medicine. Carswell took his training in Edinburgh and Glasgow, but like many other English medical students of the period, he spent some time in Paris, returning to Scotland for his M.D. After graduating, Carswell went once more to Paris to make watercolors of the large specimen collection gathered by the pathologist Jean-Philippe Louis. When the eminent anatomist J. F. Meckel declined the first Chair of Pathology at University College,

17

London, it was offered to Carswell. The governing board of the college let Carswell remain in Paris for six more months to finish a collection of drawings that amounted to more than 2,000. The drawings were of special educational value because they were available for viewing by students and physicians who did not have access to the original specimens or who could not recall their fine points.

Carswell's color drawings were refined enough in texture to differentiate one pathological state of tissue from another. Mastery of line and color was a useful accomplishment for physicians and especially for pathologists during the early nineteenth century. The list of others who illustrated their own accounts includes several who gave their names to specific anatomical features or diseases: Richard Bright, Wilhelm His, John and Charles Bell, Thomas Hodgkin and Jacob Henle.

In 1834 Carswell began to issue the fascicles of his *Pathological Anatomy: Illustrations of the Elementary Forms of Disease*. The word *illustrations* in the title was meant to be taken literally: each fascicle contains a number of colorful lithographs based on Carswell's drawings. The 12 fascicles that completed the book by 1838 were organized according to Carswell's own division of "elementary forms of disease" derived from the French tissue classification: inflammation, analogous tissues, atrophy, hypertrophy, pus, mortification, hemorrhage, softening, melanoma, carcinoma and tubercle.

During his French medical education, Carswell learned the pathology developed by Xavier Bichat late in the previous century. For Bichat and his followers, tissues (and not organs) were the fundamental components of life. Certain distinct colors and textures of tissue were diagnostic of certain diseases. Carswell made watercolors of the tissues of dead bodies to preserve their distinctive disease states more accurately than specimens in preservatives could show. The printmaking technique of lithography, invented in Germany in the 1790s, was an excellent vehicle for reproducing the critical features of the watercolors in multiple copies.

Numerous sources place the first depiction of MS lesions in Carswell's published atlas. When I examined the fascicles in the archives of the University of California–San Francisco's library, I did not know where the plate showing MS was located. The library's collection of fascicles was not complete, and thus I could not even be sure that this plate would be among those I was able to consult. I carefully turned the brittle folio pages of the inflammation, analogous tissues and atrophy sections until I came to a lithograph (Atrophy Plate IV, fig. 4) of a spinal cord with pons, brushed at intervals down its entire length with a chilling dove gray, with remains of the yellowish-brown ink that once marked those places. The paper texture, folio size and color gave the lithograph more immediacy than an anatomical photograph.

Lesions of spinal white matter with this appearance are likely to be hardened areas, or plaques of MS. Carswell's written description, though it contains little clinical information, establishes other points of MS pathology. Even the use of the word *lesion* demonstrates Carswell's French antecedents: for his mentor Louis and for his students, the lesion, a characteristic disruption of tissue, was the disease itself. In showing a new lesion, Carswell was showing a new disease.

> I have met with two cases of a remarkable lesion of the spinal cord accompanied with atrophy. One of the patients was under the care of Mons. Louis, in the Hospital of La Pitié, and the other under the care of Mons. Dhomel, in the Hospital of La Charité, both of them affected with paralysis. I did not see either of the patients, but I could not ascertain that there was anything in the character of the paralysis or the history of the cases, calculated to throw any light on the nature of the lesion found in the spinal cord. I have represented the appearances found in one of these cases in Plate IV, fig. 4, in which the pons Varolii was also affected, and which convey an accurate idea of the physical characters of the lesion. In this case a distinct portion of the cord was affected with softening, which of itself would no doubt have accounted for the paralysis; but in the other case there was no other lesion present than that to which I allude, to which the paralysis could be attributed. The anterior surface of the spinal column presented a number of spots, from a quarter of an inch to half an inch in breadth, of an irregular form, of a yellowish brown color, smooth, glossy, without vascularity or any alteration in the colour or consistence of the surrounding medullary substance. The medullary substance thus affected was very firm, somewhat transparent and atrophied. At the root of the medulla oblongata, these changes occupied the whole breadth of both the medullary fasciculus to the extent of half an inch in breadth from above downwards. Further down, they were confined to distinct spots on each fasciculus, and several of the same kind, but smaller, occupied the pons Varolii. The depth to which the medullary substance was affected in this manner varied from half a line to three or four lines, and on dividing the cord, it seemed to penetrate as far as the gray substance.

These patients had died at two of the Paris hospitals that would figure further in the history of MS. Carswell saw the lesions as an aspect of the atrophy or wasting through loss of circulatory nutrition he observed in the medullary substance surrounding them. They were remarkable in their spread over the white matter of the pons and the medulla oblongata where the brain joins the spinal column and the tracts (fasciculi) that form the spinal column. In his section on analogous tissues, those pathologies that resemble normal tissues found elsewhere in the body, Carswell detailed the cartiliginous transformation of the spinal column and, in one of his most dramatic prints, illustrated the branching, threadlike arachnoid (spidery) plaques. Unlike the long arachnoid roots of spinal hardening, however, the yellow-brown lesions occupied hardened areas and were nearly transparent. They were not like atrophies found anywhere else in the body.

The relationship between the lesion and the paralysis, which is the only clinical information he had on the disease of the patients, is established for only one of the two cases. The other case was afflicted with a softening of the spinal column, which for Carswell was a separate syphilitic pathology also likely to induce paralysis. He gave no details of brain pathology in either of the two patients.

Carswell's pathology of these lesions raised them to notice by contrast with other morbid changes in the spine. This was pathological anatomy given in greater detail than before, in color and with a large number of varied new cases, many more of them cerebral and spinal. Any anatomist examining an autopsy could at least equate lesions discovered with these illustrations and draw a further connection with any symptoms recorded.

Though he made his drawings from autopsies, Carswell isolated the affected parts as if they were prepared specimens: his spines are cleared of distracting nerves, and his brains are cut to display their abscesses and tumors. His prints are of the elementary tissue forms of disease more than of organs, vessels or other anatomical features. The yellow-brown spinal lesions (not given a name) entered into the iconography of the pathologist as far as Carswell could provide it. The size and fineness of the lithographs guaranteed that the book would not have any more editions, but those factors also made it memorable and worth consulting wherever it might be found, a traveling museum.

Carswell himself finished his life's work with the completion of his atlas in 1838 and thereafter served as a medical consultant to kings (the exiled Louis-Philippe of France and King Leopold of Belgium) as well as performing charity work. He died in 1857, possibly of chronic pulmonary tuberculosis, which he had also illustrated in one of his plates.

Virtually concurrent with Carswell's *Pathological Anatomy* fascicles, the French anatomist Jean Cruveilhier was issuing a series of his own. An old, typed librarian's card (a vanishing source of information) accompanying his works stated:

> Jean Cruveilhier (1791–1873). Son of a military surgeon, he was sent to Dupuytren. His first experience with dissections (and probably with Dupuytren's awful disposition) upset him so that he left medicine and tried to enter the priesthood. His father, a military surgeon, dragged him back and insisted he continue with medicine. Fortunately, he became fascinated with anatomy and pathology and devoted the rest of his life to the study of them. He did not use the microscope and made errors which later were corrected by Virchow.

The conditions for learning and teaching anatomy in Cruveilhier's Paris were ghastly. The composer Hector Berlioz, at first a medical student, wrote in his *Memoirs* of fleeing the anatomical theater in dread when he saw the scattered collection of human body parts and the vermin feeding on them. At the persuasions of a friend, he returned and soon was tossing a piece of an arm to a nearby rat. Perhaps this experience helped Berlioz evoke scenes of gallows and hell in his music.

Cruveilhier controlled his alarm at anatomy by taking notes and making careful drawings of the anatomical parts. He published an unillustrated *Essai sur l'anatomie pathologique en général* (2 vols., 1816). During the years between that publication and his *Anatomie pathologique* (1829–42), he gathered material from autopsies and dissections.

The principle of his pathological anatomy, as he describes it in the preface added with the completion of the book in 1835, was to draw the diseased body segments fresh from the specimen corpses as they presented themselves. Professional lithographers, named in the preface, made the prints directly from the specimens or from Cruveilhier's drawings. The fascicles of the text were issued as they were created and eventually came to fill two elephant folio volumes. In some editions they were bound in the order they were received; in other editions they were arranged according to organ or disease, with the lithographs interleaved with the written clinical descriptions. Cruveilhier eventually issued an index, by affected organ, which was bound into the final published edition. Dates given in the text spread from 1829 to 1842 even though the title page was printed in 1835.

For many cases, Cruveilhier provides a case history and clinical notes linking one case with another. Like Carswell, he was investigating the natural history of disease, but he had more contact with the living patient before death and dissection. I came to Cruveilhier's atlas aware that MS cases had been illustrated there: Charcot says so in his brief history of MS and even gives the location of the relevant cases (Charcot 1892: vol. 1, 190).

What seems to have excited some national sentiments of rivalry was Charcot's announcement that "sclérose en plaques" was depicted first by Cruveilhier in his "admirable book that should be consulted by all those who wish to avoid making secondhand discoveries." Charcot then referred to Carswell's atrophy case as another, later example.

In his 1835 preface, Cruveilhier lists a large number of recent and contemporary pathological anatomy texts, several of them dealing with brain and spinal-cord pathology. He singles out Carswell's for special praise, but he does not show any awareness of the new type of lesion Carswell described or other descriptions of the same in his own or other texts. In going to Carswell and then Cruveilhier for the earliest MS descriptions I am already following Charcot's lead and accepting the history he writes, as initiated by Cruveilhier, whom he honors as a master.

Between Cruveilhier and Charcot, a small cadre of well-situated European clinicians was able to distinguish a new tissue pathology visible only in autopsy, depict specimens in telling detail and fix the symptoms with a label linking them to the pathology.

What makes the nascent MS field of definition different from others is its remarkable (a popular word in English and French describing the lesions) appearance just at the time, the 1830s, when and in the place, Paris, where the method to detect it, the clinical-anatomical method of linking symptoms to pathological anatomy, had reached fruition. MS forms from the precise link between symptoms and pathology and opens the still-unanswered question of causation. If MS didn't exist, exponents of the method might have needed to invent it.

Charcot locates Cruveilhier's MS descriptions in fascicles 22 and 23 of the *Anatomie pathologique*, but a thorough search of text and plates does not lead to any pictures of MS lesions or details of MS symptoms. In fascicle 32, the figures of plate 2 initially raise a possibility of MS, but the clinical text does not give symptoms. The most likely instance is shown in fascicle 38, plate 5, a spinal cord lined irregularly with dove-gray patches (in the same shade as Carswell's).

This plate shows the significant remains of Josephine Paget, 38 years old, who was in bed 16 of the St. Joseph ward of La Charité on May 4, 1840. She had bronchitis when Cruveilhier first examined her and was considerably weakened, though she could hold herself upright and walk with a little help, all the while shaking on her legs. Her left leg was a good deal weaker than her right. She had difficulty picking up a needle. After 18 months, Cruveilhier found her weaker still. She dropped her bread, her spoon, anything she tried to hold. Her fingers were fattened as if she had "ants," that is, joint mice, an arthritic condition.

The doctor diagnosed an illness of the spinal tissue and, since there was no serious pain, a paralysis due to fluid compression of the spinal nerves. By March 9, 1841, she was feeling pain on her left side and greater numbness, though she retained the ability to move her fingers. Her skin had lost feeling, but her muscles were highly reactive. Cruveilhier was sure that this was an acute spinal arachnitis, an infection of the arachnoid layer of the spine. He prescribed regular baths and some purgatives. She complained of feeling a constriction like a belt or a log resting on different parts of her body. On March 12 the pain had grown so severe that she cried out, "Dogs are gnawing at me." She died, suffocated by bronchial blockage, at 9 A.M., March 20.

The autopsy showed pleurisy of the left lung. At first glance the spinal column itself seemed unblemished, but on closer examination Cruveilhier discovered that the nervous tissue had succumbed to a grayish degeneration. On the spinal white matter separated from the gray jacket, the degeneration took the form of patches (this is the subject of plate 5). The patches were superficial but reached a certain depth of the gray matter. They were denser than the spinal cord itself, and they replaced the spinal matter, precisely filling in any gaps without forming a line. There was no other morbid tissue, though some few medullary fibers escaped degeneration and showed white in the gray patches.

Cruveilhier records that he had not detected the pleurisy, the result of residing in a humid place (the hospital?). Even auscultation (listening to the lungs through a horn applied to the chest) had not disclosed it to him. Possibly if she had complained of being fastened with a corset rather than a belt, he would have recognized the underlying problem.

"It remains to determine," Cruveilhier reflected in his final note, "how the gray degeneration of the spine comes about. It is not an apopleptic [stroke] lesion. There is nothing in this gray tissue that resembles a scar. Might it be one of the numerous effects that result from a phlegmatic attack? Only [with] further observations aimed at studying how this remarkable lesion develops can this question of the lesion's origins be settled."

In terms sometimes resembling Carswell's, Cruveilhier set the agenda for the histological study of the MS lesion, a study that would not actually be taken up for some decades and not by his French successors. Cruveilhier also set down the first clinical history that can be identified as MS from anatomical materials. As an exponent and patron of the *méthode clinico-anatomique*, he correlated the autopsy with the symptoms and speculated on the role of the lesions, which he saw as the underlying cause of Josephine Paget's condition, though she actually succumbed to pleurisy. She may have distracted him from the diagnosis of pleurisy by saying she felt a belt rather than a corset, but she managed to convey one important description of MS symptoms in the process.

A careful chronological study shows that Carswell published the very first pictorial depiction of MS (Compston 1988:1251). That the two spine pictures resemble each other strongly and, along with Carswell's lack of a case history, raise the possibility that Carswell and Cruveilhier were describing the same patient. They were contemporaries in Paris and Lyon, were likely to have been acquainted and may even have examined the same unusual cases. But Josephine Paget lived until March 20, 1841, and Carswell's atlas was complete in 1838. There were at least two different cases of MS anatomized at Paris or Lyon hospitals between the early 1830s and 1841.

There may have been some earlier than that. In his *Morbid Anatomy of the Human Brain* (1829), Robert Hooper published a lithograph that might show the features of MS. But the plate is unlabeled and is not attached to a clinical history. It could illustrate any number of cerebral conditions. Hooper's unpublished plates are likewise not specific enough to show distinct MS plaques.

In 1831, in the second volume of his *Reports of Medical Cases*, Richard Bright described several cases that have some features of MS, most notably

Case CCCIII (1831:604), a 24-year-old woman with a three-year history of varying weakness and numbness in her lower limbs. These cases were descriptions of the symptoms of the living; Bright was unable to record or illustrate postmortem results. Near as others came, it was left for Carswell to provide the first link between the symptoms and the pathological appearance of MS.

In 1824 the young anatomist Charles Ollivier d'Angers published *De la moelle épinière et de ses maladies* (On the spinal column and its illnesses), in which d'Angers described the symptomatic history of a man then in his early forties. This man had good health until the age of 17 but then began to have spells of tiredness. When he was 20, his right foot became weak, and five years later his lower limbs were weak and numb, though there were sporadic improvements. By the age of 30, he was walking with a cane. Hot spa waters, he found, aggravated his condition with an especially acute loss of coordination in his right leg and clumsiness in both hands. He suffered retention of urine and had to press on his abdomen to empty his bowels. When he touched his thigh with his paretic right hand, he felt a "galvanic" shock running through his body (the earliest description of what was later called Lhermitte's sign). His speech was labored. Yet during the years after the symptoms began, he did not suffer impairment of intellect nor did he lose his cheerfulness of disposition. This man was still very much alive when Ollivier d'Angers wrote down his case, and given the circumstances of clinical encounters with those not critically ill, Ollivier d'Angers was unable to follow the case or perform an autopsy.

John Spillane, in his history of neurology, refers to this as the "best documented early account of what was probably multiple sclerosis" he had encountered (Spillane 1981:205). "Probable" is the second of the three grades of likelihood recognized in the present-day diagnosis of MS. The case of Ollivier d'Angers wins that grade because of the presence of changing lower limb and speech symptoms, together with a heat reaction and the surprising presence of a Lhermitte's sign. Among other possibilities, these signs could also be indicative of neurosyphilis, and Ollivier d'Angers himself appears to be suggesting that. The particular development of the symptoms does make a case for MS. Because it was Cruveilhier and not Ollivier d'Angers who taught the next generation of French pathological anatomists, Cruveilhier was remembered as the describer of *sclérose en plaques*—though more defensively than clearly as Charcot's mistaken reference shows.

Among the many pathological anatomies and case history compilations published during these years, and the many more still in manuscript, how many equally suggestive early MS examples are there to uncover? If there are, they are likely to be vague pictures or isolated symptom accounts. There are centuries of pictures and descriptions of what might or might not be MS. Yet it is unlikely that there is another that joins a graphic picture of pathological anatomy with a case history like the one Cruveilhier set down. Josephine Paget was the first named person to die of complications related to multiple sclerosis, and Cruveilhier was the first person to leave a picture of the evidence.

3

Two MS Lives:
Heine and d'Esté

Guessing backward in time about the diseases of illustrious people is a common pastime of medicine. The search for victims of multiple sclerosis before multiple sclerosis was an established diagnosis has hit on two figures of the early nineteenth century, widely different from each other yet sharing some similarities. Apart from the symptoms themselves, it is suggestive that both came down with their disease at the same time that the first MS cases were being described in France, Germany and England.

The great German poet Heinrich Heine died in 1856, at age 59, after about 25 years of suffering. Augustus d'Esté, the English military officer and pretender to a dukedom, died in 1848, at 54 years old, having suffered his first signs some 22 years earlier.

Whereas the early cases of presumed multiple sclerosis were recorded as pathological anatomy with some clinical information, and scarcely a name to them, both Heine and d'Esté recorded their own lives and symptoms, and neither was subjected to an autopsy. If women are indeed more prone to multiple sclerosis than men, it continues to be true even today that men are more likely to write about their condition, though the proportion is evening out. Literate men of position in literary and social worlds, both these men craved the public assertion of an identity that had been denied them, Heine his Jewishness and his Germanness and d'Esté his succession to his father's ducal rank and royal pedigree. Neither wrote exclusively to describe his illness, but each wrote down enough details to encourage later speculation.

The diagnoses of Heine's troubles have varied over the years. He himself seemed convinced that he had neurosyphilis, and this has been affirmed by a succession of medical biographers (Critchley 1969). Hereditary disease, porphyria, stroke and spinal degeneration have also been suggested.

As a student, Heine suffered from severe headaches. In letters written in 1831 he described brief paralytic episodes in his eyelids and two fingers. His vision became disturbed, weakening and then recovering in alternation. By the late 1830s he had the syphilitic's dread of incipient blindness. In 1843 the left side of his face was paralyzed, and a numbness spread down the left side of his body. Heine was not isolated in his illness. The death of his uncle Solomon, both a mainstay and an antagonist, precipitated a breakdown. In 1848 Heine had a complete collapse and was left paralyzed in the lower extremities, buried alive in his "mattress tomb" until his death exactly eight years later. "They were eight years of unremitting torture, during which he produced some of his greatest and most moving work" (Pawel 1995:6).

Heine's biographer Ernst Pawel discredits the syphilis judgment: Heine never suffered the emotional and mental instability of advanced tabes dorsalis (spinal syphilis with a distinct set of symptoms). After adding amyotrophic lateral sclerosis (ALS) and muscular dystrophies (but not multiple sclerosis) to the disease possibilities, Pawel declares the disease question to be academic.

Heine's contemporary doctors treated his symptoms directly, subjecting him to medications and blistering procedures that increased his suffering. He became addicted to morphine. None of these physicians left a contemporary record of the poet's physical condition, and he does not seem to have come into contact with any of the clinical anatomists maturing their craft in Paris while he was dying there. The German émigré ophthalmologist Julius Sichel did treat Heine's eyes from 1837 on, and E.H. Jellinek (1990:518) speculates that Sichel's (1852, vol. 1) unnamed case of a 45-year-old man with optic disc atrophy compatible with recovery of sight was Heine. That ophthalmoscopic piece is perhaps the only medical record of Heine.

Heine first mentioned his eye problems and his consultation with Sichel in a letter written from Paris, on September 15, 1837, to Julius Campe. On March 24, 1839, he wrote to the composer Giacomo Meyerbeer that he was afraid of going blind and that Sichel had advised him to reduce his amount of work. But even in 1844 he was still writing to correspondents, such as Karl Marx, that his eyes were worsening. He had reached a state of discomfort that made it seem he was always getting worse because he improved intermittently. Throughout, he was subjected to contemporary medical treatments aimed at alleviating the symptoms. In a letter postmarked Passy, June 12, 1848, "I can drag on this way for another dozen years. The last two weeks I have been so completely paralyzed that I have to be carried like a child; my legs are as if made of cotton-wool. My eyes are wretched. But my heart is whole and my brain and stomach are in good condition" (Heine 1948:453).

He wrote to Heinrich Laube from Paris, on January 25, 1850:

> For the last year and three-quarters I have been tortured day and night by the most horrible agonies, confined to my bed, and paralyzed in all

my members. Incessant cramps, most insufferable spasms, practically total blindness — a calamity rarely met with in the annals of human suffering — an unheard-of, horrible, insane calamity! I suffer from the most terrible hopelessness and spiritual torments, but I bear these, as I do the physical ones, with a tranquillity I would never have believed I was capable of. My brain has grown weak because I lie constantly on my back and because of overdoses of dulling opiates — but it is not a total ruin, and I hope to preserve some of my clarity to the very end — which, between you and me — is not far off [Heine 1948:461].

The sources on Heine's health are his own writing and some contemporary drawings that illustrate his posture and facial aspects. From these, Jellinek (1990) and Stenager (1996) contest the compatibility of Heine's symptoms with neurosyphilis: his symptoms were relapsing and remitting, whereas the blindness or the strokes resulting from syphilitic infections of spine and arteries are without recovery. And Heine complained of some facial palsies that might have been due to unusual multiple sclerosis lesions of cranial nerves.

All commentators emphasize that Heine's poetry transcended his sickness for the poet himself and for his readers (Kadish and Gadoth 1995). Heine achieved this transcendence not by ignoring his condition but by using his disease state (in the later poetry) as an expressive tool and a source of metaphor. His image of himself as "ich arme unbegrabene Leiche" (I the poor unburied corpse) (unpublished poems, "Mathilde," in Pawel 1995:266–67) is a reference to his state of paralysis lying abed those many years and also to the corpse exposed to public mourning for the singing of the Kaddish. Only here the singer is the corpse himself.

From among the numbers of biblical and mythological figures he could have chosen to represent his condition, Heine chose Lazarus more decisively than Job or Faust. Lazarus was the hope of personal resurrection and the triumph of faith over death and decay. As a Jewish convert of convenience to Catholicism, Heine chose the image of a man who (for Christians) had died in Judaism and been reborn in Christianity, but the renewal of faith he felt during his struggle with the severe attacks was not a desperate or fanatical embrace of any religion. His letters confirming the stories of his disease are also protests against being judged a zealot. His Lazarus was the man on the mat always about to be relieved of his paralysis by a renewal of faith. Whether he had MS or not, his waiting for rebirth was a spiritual response to chronic disease, a response often repeated in MS history.

In the supplement to his poem "Lazarus" published in *Poems of 1853 and 1854*, he gives a portrait of himself as the afflicted man.

> Es hatte mein Haupt die schwartze Frau
> Zärtlich ans Herz geschlossen;
> Ach! meine Haare wurden grau,
> Wo ihre Tränen geflossen.

Sie küßte mich lahm, sie küßte mich krank,
Sie küßte mir blind die Augen;
Das Mark aus meinem Rückgrat trank
Ihr Mund mit wildem Saugen.

Mein Leib ist jetzt ein Leichnam, worin
Der Geist ist eingekerkert —
Manchmal wird ihm unwirsch zu Sinn,
Er tobt und rast und berserkert.

Ohnmächtige Flüche! Dein schlimmster Fluch
Wird keine Fliege töten.
Ertrage die Schickung, und versuch,
Gelinde zu flennen, zu beten.

(The dark woman took my head
sweetly to her breast;
And turned my locks of hair all gray,
wherever her tears fell.

She kissed me lame, she kissed me sick,
she kissed my eyes all blind;
The strength from my spine she drank
with wild, abandoned thirsting.

Now my body is a corpse, wherein
my spirit is imprisoned —
Often it loses all sense,
it shakes and rages and rattles.

Powerless curses! Your strongest shriek
Can hardly shake a fly.
Tolerate what you've earned, and seek,
peace in whining, and in prayer.)

After the insult of translation, I might as well add a matter-of-fact interpretation of the references in this poem. The "dark woman" could be syphilis, a word that Heine himself never used. She is an image of the female absorption of male energy, an act assumed to precede and activate the disease. His energy to move and act in the realm of affairs having been lost, his *Geist* can only rage like a chained prisoner, but his words no longer have any effect. From the male power to love and give out potent words Heine has fallen back to complaint and a search for inner peace, but not of self-examination. He was less concerned with examining the physical details of his illness than with finding a way to live through it.

Further along in the same set of poems he tells of the "*Tummelplatz*" (revel) that the ancient gods and phantoms make of his skull at night and how after a night of this sport, the poet's "*Leichenhand*" (corpse hand) tries to write it down. This is Heine's pathological anatomy. The tumultuous interior he must show through writing, but the instrument itself is numb. The inscribing devices developed to record the motions of trembling hands would not have satisfied Heine because the element of volition was missing from the marks made.

One of Heine's written fantasies was of the British inventor who made a mechanical man. The automaton operated so well that it recognized it lacked a soul and began to beg its maker for one. The inventor fled abroad, and his invention pursued him. This was the origin of the two figures met everywhere: "a part of the English people weary of their mechanical existence, demand a soul-another, appalled by this demand, flee here and there. But neither of them can stay at home."

Heine's craving for release from suffering gives unsentimental poignancy of his own anguish worsened by the seeming reprieves. He repeats stock phrases about being tired of life and shows that he really means them. At the same time his sensitivity to earthly things has become a discomfort: the red flowers he cannot bear to see or smell are intolerable in themselves and for the memories they evoke. What he enjoyed most in life no longer quickens him. He is ready to make his final testament and hand down his pain and debility to his enemies as he makes his escape.

Heine was not completely absorbed by his illness even at the very end. It would be a disservice to read his life in its terms, even as a noble, anxious resistance against debility and failure. Besides some evidence of an early, eminent case of the disease, Heine gives a rare look at one person's response to its peculiar state (shared with ALS): paralysis accompanied by mental lucidity. For his own comfort and in his writing, he drew on older images of the soul within the body and of the dying man. For Heine, the disease was a prolonged deathbed from which he might yet rise again. He expresses the disappointed hope of an intermittently recovering but ever-degenerating body. This forms an imagery of desire and need that is remote from the physicians' evolving description of MS.

One of the results of the German blockade of the British isles during 1940–41 was a shortage of paper, and there was a drive to gather waste paper for conversion into pulp. During the search of one of the London Sector hospitals, a number of manuscripts were discovered; one of them, found with a collection of letters, diaries and account books, was presented to the Royal College of Physicians for its medical interest. A fellow of the college, Dr. Douglas Firth, soon read before the History of Medicine Section excerpts from this manuscript, entitled by its author "The Case of Augustus d'Esté." The excerpts were published in *Proceedings of the Royal Society of Medicine* (Firth 1941).

Firth prepared the entire manuscript for publication, a process delayed by the war, and he had seen the book through the press and the final proofs when he died suddenly. The tiny book (Firth 1948) appeared 100 years after its subject died. In his preface, Firth refers to it as "possibly the earliest clinical account of disseminated sclerosis, albeit written by a layman." Firth's book remedies d'Esté's lack of medical judgment, with Firth writing and annotating Augustus d'Esté's personal history to underline symptoms. As befit his station, d'Esté consulted and was treated by a number of eminent medical men of the day. Firth uses that opportunity to study medical practices and personalities of the time and to gossip a little on royal family politics.

Circumstances permit a more than usual scrutiny of the medical history of the child, Augustus, born to Lady Augusta Murray and Prince Augustus Frederick, the sixth son of George III, king of England, on January 13, 1794. Prince Augustus had been touring the continent seeking relief from his asthma when he met Lady Augusta in Italy. Their clandestine marriage so enraged the king, who was determined to control alliances within his own family, that he ordered his son home. Prince Augustus returned but then married Lady Augusta openly and legally. The king had the marriage annulled, and the child, Augustus Frederick, became illegitimate and not eligible for baptism in a Christian rite. His mother survived a birthing infection and took great care of her son, noting his ailments and her attending physician's advice in a notebook. From this record it is obvious that the baby not only suffered from common childhood infections and infestations but also, in keeping with his father's and other relatives' history, had bouts of allergy, St. Anthony's fire and eczema of the scalp. Though it may or may not be related, we should recall (which Firth doesn't) George III's affliction, thought later to be porphyria. When Lady Augusta's father tried to press his daughter's case in an audience with the king, the meeting ended with them both referring to the other's children as "bastards." Porphyria has limited value as an explanation of this behavior.

That Prince Augustus left his wife when he became a royal duke was a severe disappointment to her, because it meant that her son had less chance of a succession to his father's and (possibly, even) his grandfather's estate. She referred to herself as the "Duchess of Sussex" and her son as "Prince Augustus" for the rest of her life. This was the immediate basis for her son's quest for enfranchisement, which he pursued with Parliament after the king himself was dead and with his own father.

Lady Augusta's extreme solicitude and hopes for her son are expressed in her letters urging him to remain healthy and in account-book entries referring to payments made to doctors treating "my Boy" for measles and chicken pox and to her expenditures supporting his growing self-indulgence. His father gave him a family name (Este) that would suggest no royal aspirations and tried unsuccessfully to remove him from his mother's influence. Sent to join an army regiment as an officer, Augustus kept a journal in which he praised the virtues of tinned "bouilli" beef (a source of poisonous lead leaching into the food from the solder) and exhibited what Firth considers "an abnormal mental condition." In the journal, Augustus records several incidents in which he embroiled himself with other men over trivial matters and then agonized about his own behavior. With this, Firth ends his exposé of the "psychological traumata" of d'Esté's childhood and adolescence, "which may be of interest as aetiological factors in disseminated sclerosis."

The manuscript entitled "The Case of Augustus d'Esté," written in installments in various handwritings including Augustus' and that of his sister, was probably begun in 1830 and ended in 1844. The "case" of the title is both Augustus' case of his illness and his case for the succession to his father's titles; in Firth's hands it becomes a medical case history, one that, in fact, he found useful to illustrate diagnostic points to medical students. In 1822, when Augustus was in Scotland for the funeral of a relative, his eyes were "so attacked that when fixed upon minute objects indistinctness of vision was the consequence," though he was not aware of this until he attempted to read or cut his pen. In 1825 he sometimes saw "imagined spots" floating before his eyes.

Late 1827 was the first serious crisis in his health, one most suggestive of the disease. On October 17 he recorded a "torpor or indistinctness" about the temple of his left eye, this evolving into a confusion of sight and then into double vision. Dr. Kissock suggested it was due to an excess of the humor bile, and Augustus was "blooded" from the temple by leeches, given a purge to make him vomit and then blooded again from the arm. His sight improved. "Now a new disease began to shew itself: every day I found *gradually* (by slow degrees) my strength leaving me: I could clearly perceive each succeeding day that I went up and down the staircase with greater difficulty. When I slapped myself sharply on the loins (though only momentary the effect) yet for the time it increased my strength."

This horseman's response to the failure of his limbs to function was not very successful. His strength began to return when Dr. Kent made him eat beefsteaks twice a day and drink wine (to restore his energy) and had him rubbed on the back with an opium liniment for an hour twice a day. He was able to travel to Rome and ride out on horseback most days, though he could not run as before and he could not dance at all. Discontinuing the brush rubbing, he had his servant slap him with open hand toward the sacrum.

In the following entries Augustus chronicled his attacks and his treatments over the next 16 years. He was unable to follow former pursuits, such as chamois hunting in the Alps, with his former vigor, but the mountain air at least restored his strength enough to permit long mountain walks. He experienced retention of urine during military maneuvers and theorized that this was caused both by want of sufficient muscular force to expel the water and by an irritation of the bladder itself. A surgeon passing a bougie (a metal cylinder) into his urethra broke a membranous obstruction, leading to some relief, but Augustus, later considering the obstruction's return as a possible explanation for the "deficiency of wholesome vigour" that he experienced in a liaison with a young woman, doubted there ever was an obstruction. When he experienced a "dreadful lowness of spirits," he blamed it on the valerian he was taking, the heat in his residence and his habit of smoking more than usual.

Through sea bathings and galvanic treatments, Augustus pursued both his lost health and his dukedom. His setbacks in his ducal quest became one more symptomatic irritation amid the numbness, pains and travails of long carriage rides about Europe. He was especially afflicted with a numbness of the lower back and thighs. Whenever he was able to take exercise, either walking or horseback riding, he noticed an improvement.

In 1842 Priesznitz, the owner of the spa at Gräfenburg, Hanover, told him that his infirmity originated in the nerves. After the eccentric and critical physician Samuel Dickson dosed him with prescriptions (given in the text) containing strychnine and silver nitrate, he had his first serious attack of vertigo, became "as sick as a dog" and yet rose with the assurance that he never once fainted or lost consciousness. As he retired from Brighton to escape "the keenness of the Air," he consulted John Scott in London and received milder prescriptions as well as an exercise regimen: "to ride on horseback every day … to walk out of doors every hour." In telling of this, he recorded his own belief that "the exercise of volition is indispensable to the restoration of muscular power," thus reflecting the doctrine that muscular debility was due to will not entering the muscles. By December 1843, in Brighton again, because of the "searching quality of the Sea Air" he was gradually becoming less capable of taking exercise.

In answer to his appeal for a consultation, John Scott sent Dr. J. R. Farre, who read over Augustus' case book, interrogated him and together with Mr. Scott (who, as a surgeon, was not "doctor") formed the opinion that Augustus' disease was "Paraplegia and is either Active or Passive, Functional or Organic." The two consultants not only offered a full medical name and a course for Augustus' troubles but also proposed a treatment plan. Declaring that all healing comes from a change in circulation, the doctors placed responsibility for improvement with the patient himself, according to an age-old regimen: "He must not offend in either the quantity or the quality of his food; he must not exceed his physical limits in the exertions either of his body or of his mind; but above all he must guard against the emotions of his mind, which instantly perturb the actions of his heart." Apart from professional caution against patient disobedience, this plan takes into account the excesses and stresses of Augustus' life and uses a vague medical rationale to try to get him to mend his ways. But in early 1844 Augustus found his stamina decreasing and could not comply fully with the instructions. Always seeking a pharmaceutical cause of his declines, he discovered that a small amount of mercury in one of his prescriptions may have brought about a heavy languor that "floors" him. From this point he tried the Brighton airs and electricity again several times, concluding that they both worsened his condition. He sought the advice of Dr. Augustus Bozzi Granville, who was healed of a similar infirmity by taking the waters at Bath. He did not follow Granville's advice, however; instead, under other doctors, one of whom died during the course of treatment, he went through the old "piano" routine, which did him no good. In the midst of this, he received very unfavorable news from the House of Lords committee considering his claim. After the honors conferred on the Duchess of Inverness, his father's legal wife, Augustus "remained NEGLECTED—in the MIRE," which might almost have been a description of his treatment at Bath.

Whether following a medical system or not, Augustus sought the right air and waters to give him health. He actually found the air in London restorative after a sojourn in the hill resort of St. Leonard's, where in addition the ankle of his left leg began to turn out at every step. He catalogued his feelings and complaints: spasms in his feet and legs, spasms while trying to sit, discomfort while lying down for any length of time. His sensation around his middle was "as if my Legs, having been out of Joint at the Thigh Sockets, had been restored to their proper places; but still were under the Influence of the Injury which they had sustained." It is not too surprising that when Dr. Edward James Seymour said there was no organic "evil" and that he had healed cases worse than this, Augustus took what Seymour prescribed—medicines containing cantharides ("Spanish fly")—which then required that he take a soothing medicine against the irritations they produced.

The last entry in his case (December 17, 1846) tells of receiving a gift of Indian moccasins, which relieve him of the turning ankle and the steel ankle-stay he had been wearing. During the remaining two years of his life Augustus kept another diary detailing further medical treatments by Dr. Seymour and chronicling his episodes of pain and spasm. On the row and column pages of an account book, he recorded his daily walks around his room, using a chronometer to time himself one round per minute and entering the total minutes in the paid column of the book (almost like a neurological pacing test). An exceptionally good time (59 minutes) he entered in red ink; a poor time (10¼ minutes or 6 minutes) he preceded with an "Alas." He was aging rapidly, becoming deaf and so spastic that he could walk only with the support of a servant or by sitting himself in his "chair on wheels." There is no contemporary information on his final illness other than the month and year of his death, December 1848. Firth concludes his own book by praising the clinical accuracy of d'Esté's account while reflecting on how curious it was that the disease was not better known in that time. Firth notes, "As Charcot himself considered the disease something of a curiosity, it may well be that it was as rare when Augustus d'Esté embarked upon his personal history as it is common today."

Augustus d'Esté can sound like a hypochondriac or chronic complainer. Rather than transcending his pain, as Heine did, with lyricism and humor, d'Esté seems languishing and agitated, always trying to move about. The disease was a convenient metaphor for d'Esté's life struggle to gain, or regain, his estate. His life became known as a clinical example of disseminated sclerosis only through Firth's interpretation of his diaries. Before that, d'Esté was a minor figure in English dynastic history, an illegitimate son of a royal duke trying to keep from falling into the minor nobility. As a result of arriving in medical consciousness in the twentieth century, and in a time when the British, reeling from a devastating war, needed to look to their unique monarchy and its traditions, d'Esté's case never has been judged as Heine's was in his own time and afterward — as something not quite so "clean," as advanced syphilis or tabes dorsalis. Most subsequent writers appear willing to take Douglas Firth's word on the matter and to treat d'Esté monolithically as the "first case of disseminated sclerosis." A more cautious assessment of the case would probably label it one of the earliest personal accounts of chronic neurological disease, of which MS eventually became the model.

The aspects of d'Esté's case reflect his struggle against the loss of control and the remedies that he spontaneously tried and his physicians recommended. With his doctors, d'Esté shared a view of which sensations were healthful and which procedures were likely to be curative. The doctors could constantly play on his desire for treatment and offer instructions that might be taken as the cause of any improvement. The fluctuating but, in the long run, downward trend of d'Esté's health created opportunities for speculative treatments that recur in the history of MS. Recently a celebrity with multiple sclerosis recommended horseback riding at a particular ranch in the American Southwest. Cantharides and substances like them are always breaking out in the MS pharmacopoeia.

Heine and d'Esté are the earliest full lives that may have been multiple sclerosis lives, whatever else they meant in their day. Many of the themes of their lives continue in other and later lives. Their stature kept them from becoming cases, mere examples of the disease in the custody of the medical profession. The effectiveness of their understanding and the resultant treatments are made all too plain in the chronicle of a privileged patient like d'Esté. But his life has come to attention only because a doctor examined his writings and made him into a case.

People not situated to receive medical care may have been less subject to the tortures that d'Esté and, to some extent, Heine went through under the pretense of treatment. Later historians have even claimed that the diet of the wealthy or their access to dental fillings and medicines compounded with mercury made them more likely than poorer people to develop MS damage in the central nervous system. What underlying damage Heine or d'Esté suffered we will never know. Neither was anatomized after death. Even in this era of medically interested exhumations of poets, tsars and presidents, no one has opened their graves to have a look.

Postmortem examinations of the body's insides were reserved for the exe-cuted criminals and abandoned paupers. We know there was MS in the 1830s because a few afflicted paupers ended their lives in places such as La Charité and La Pitié in Paris, where a Cruveilhier might match spasms during life with patches discovered on the spine and brain stem of the freely opened corpse. The poet and the pretender recorded their own lives for other reasons.

Literate people examined their own lives in the early nineteenth century in a manner that might render evidence for the presence of MS. For instance, another German poet, Eduard Mörike, had a long life (1804–75) of small afflictions that can be taken as due to MS. His struggle with the rigid rules of the German church in which he was a rural minister, the domestic conflict between his wife and his sister and his own sensitivity to the world around him also influenced the course of his life. All we can do is apply our MS model to the known biography of symptoms and make a guess.

> Herr, schicke was du willt,
> Ein Liebes oder Leides!
> Ich bin vergnügt, dass beides
> Aus deinen Händen quillt...
>
> (Lord, send what you will,
> Some love or some sorrow!
> I am content, that both
> flow freely from your hand...)

4

MS Embodied

In 1833 a Göttingen university physician and lecturer named Karl Friedrich Heinrich Marx presented a Latin monograph entitled *De paralysi membrorum inferiorum* (On the paralysis of the lower limbs) before the Gottinger Gesellschaft der Wissenschaften. Marx published the paper in German in 1838, and it was hardly noticed by other physicians studying the same condition. Studies of paraplegia written by members of the Paris faculties soon after its publication did not mention it at all (Keppel Hesselink 1991a: 2440).

Marx's monograph presents cases of slowly progressive paraplegia he had seen develop in his patients over the years. Patients, he declared, usually come to the doctor when the paralysis has already become pronounced, and they attribute it to a condition of the bones, such as rheumatism, though the bone condition may be the result of the paralysis rather than its cause.

He had the opportunity to review a long symptomatic development in the case of a woman he saw first in 1824; at the age of 45, she complained of acute pains in her right knee, of eye pain and of urinary incontinence. The troubles had begun in 1823 with a loss of sensation in her feet. She was married, with seven children, and she believed that going into the children's room at night during the winter, not wearing any shoes and without a carpet on the floor, had given her a chill that "settled" into the soles of her feet. Soon she was feeling acute pains in her ankles and knees, limiting her ability to step forward or backward. This "anguish" (*"Übel"* in the patient's first-person description, which Marx quoted) spread into her right arm and hand, but it fluctuated seasonally, diminishing in springtime only to return redoubled in the summer.

The woman told Marx that she began to feel temperature changes in her foot as if warm butter were being poured over it. Cold spells were followed by warm pinpricks all over the skin surface. The bones cramped up when she tried to walk, and at night she often was wakened by leg spasms. These

39

problems didn't inhibit her from walking some distance during a visit to the city in 1827, but after that she was unable to stand erect. The left leg cramped as severely as the right, yet on examination Marx could see no signs of atrophy in the leg muscles. Walking became impossible, and arm action was seriously limited. Her speech was disturbed, though it remained sufficiently intact for her to cry out in anguish. She died in extreme pain during what appeared to be a seizure.

An autopsy performed under Marx's supervision disclosed no abnormalities in her viscera. In the white matter of the "enlarged, blood-rich spinal column" ("*vergrösserte blutreiche Rückenmarke*") were found hard patches as deep as they were wide, filled with a grayish red mass like old coagulated blood. There were similar patches about 1 × .5 cm in size distributed on the fibers leading to the cauda equinal "horse tail," the fan of nerves at the base of the spine) but not on the cauda itself. Marx did not observe comparable patches on any of the spinal nerve connections.

In Marx's judgment, the patient's troubles began with blood congestion of nerves in the white matter of the spine, which led to isolated bleeding and the formation of coagulated patches. This primary pathogenic process induced the ultimately fatal degeneration of the secondary nerve connections. Marx did not believe that the progressive debility was due to localized nerve damage; he believed it followed from a failure in the link between central and peripheral nervous systems. The pinpricks were not the result of rheumatism in the bones, as the patient thought, but were a consequence of the nerve disruption.

This pathology took a total of six years to develop and was not accompanied by muscle atrophy, which meant that the patches did not block the nerves entirely. Other, more acute cases of lower limb paralysis in which the patients did show muscle atrophy had been recorded, but like this one, these did not show any signs of dementia. Urinary and fecal incontinence and a remitting-relapsing pattern of symptoms were also characteristic of these cases. Marx did not know whether medullary patches (in the spinal matter) were present in any of these others.

Though both Carswell's and Cruveilhier's volumes were published by the time of the appearance of Marx's paper in German in 1838 (they would not have been available before his Latin paper of 1833), and though Cruveilhier's at least was in the possession of the medical faculty at Gottingen at a later date, there is no evidence that Marx saw either of them. He does not refer directly or indirectly to the "yellowish-brown lesions" or "*sclérose en isles*," references that would imply he was drawing from his British or French contemporaries.

His description of the patient's symptom course was in accordance with Hermann Boerhaave's classic compendium: setting forth the progress of the symptoms; obtaining anatomical corroboration; and forming a surmise of the internal course of events that led to the course exhibited. He singled out the spinal lesions, believing they were the result of an internal hemorrhaging and coagulation that compromised nerve flow, and he compared the symptoms with other paraplegia cases that had come to his attention. J. M. Keppel Hesselink (1991a) argues that Marx's is the first clinical description of a case of multiple sclerosis. But it was not cited in subsequent articles on paralytic diseases or MS, nor was Marx himself included in biographical dictionaries of prominent German physicians of the nineteenth century. Since the paper was unknown to practicing physicians except perhaps as a contribution to the oral repository of case comparisons that Marx refers to, it had no influence over the developing formal medical consciousness of the symptom complex and its relationship with the lesions. The same might be said of Ollivier d'Anger's even earlier clinical description (1824).

Marx lived until 1877, dying at the age of 81. His contribution was not noted in such works as Ludwig Muller's *De induratione medullae spinalis* (printed in Bonn, 1842, and reprinted in *Jaccoud* 1873: vol. 1, 330–42) or F. T. Frerichs' important summary "Über Hirnsclerose," published in *Archiv des Geschichtes der Medezin (Häsers Archiv)* in 1849 (10:334–50). Muller and Frerichs were in their turn neglected in the standard history of MS leading to Charcot, but like Marx, they seem to have represented moments of a growing communal knowledge — among practitioners — of a spinal-brain patch-symptom link possibly not syphilitic in nature. Marx's case, like Cruveilhier's, defines a moment at which both symptoms and pathology were present in the same individual. After this, focus moves to unusual tissues and deeper, and the person is lost.

Friedrich Theodor von Frerichs (1819–85) was best known during the nineteenth century for his text on liver diseases (*Über Leberkrankheiten*). His article on sclerosis of the brain appeared earlier in his career, while he was still attempting to establish himself as a practitioner. It was composed as a summation of knowledge up to that point, mentioning Cruveilhier's and several other case study articles that had appeared, as well as a number of his own cases.

Frerichs clearly understands that he is describing the same kind of lesion as his cited predecessors, but he goes beyond them in making lesions of the brain the primary focus of his attention. He does not take the long view that Marx did, watching a case develop. His patients are little more than their own remains reflecting the symptoms caused by the lesions. This emphasis on tissue rather than history gives Frerichs strong comparative resources: he is the first to establish the link between remitting-relapsing paralysis during life and the consistent presence of the lesions after death. He makes the same environmental association as Carswell and Marx, finding a humid environment likely to have initiated the tissue changes that led to the multiplication of the lesions.

Frerichs was an academic physician who moved between privatdocent and professorship posts, eventually establishing himself in Berlin. He came to specialize in the liver because that organ seemed to show degeneration that more clearly corresponded with external symptoms than did the brain or spine. Frerichs's considerations on brain sclerosis, printed in one of the first European journals devoted to the general medicine, was an early attempt to accomplish with brain diagnosis what he was later more successful in accomplishing with the liver. Frerichs's cases of brain sclerosis were exactly that: examples of hardening of cerebral tissue discovered postmortem. Judging from his descriptions, most of the cases were not MS, which is confirmed by the scant symptomatic accounts accompanying the pathology. Frerichs did not distinguish categorically between a diffuse sclerosis and a disseminated sclerosis, which he might have with more examples available. He saw all cerebral hardening as the same primary pathological process.

Frerichs's brain studies and indeed his liver work were part of German-state investigations that fit generally into the Naturphilosophie emerging from Immanuel Kant's philosophy articulated during the foregoing century. It might be possible to ally Carswell with British empiricism, Cruveilhier with Cartesian rationalism and the Germans from Marx to Frerichs with Kant, who had formed a critique of both traditions. They were all seeking to match hidden physical changes with observable symptoms.

With Frerichs, the observation that the lesions were of spinal and brain white matter but not of peripheral nerves or of other tissue became firmly established. The general nature of the lesions as a tissue phenomenon became wider knowledge in the medical schools. Frerichs was so successful in bringing forth the essence of what was known, and those after him were so consistent in following the program of which his work was part, that the British historian of medicine Charles Singer cited Frerichs's article as the first complete clinical analysis of multiple sclerosis (Singer 1925:169). Singer may have been following the judgment of the medical bibliographers Garrison and Morton, for whom Frerichs's paper was the first significant study of MS. Garrison and Singer saw the development of medicine as the triumph of sharper, brighter knowledge over quackery and superstition, and Frerichs certainly supplied the MS instance for their collection.

At the same time that Singer was writing, German historians of medicine seemed unaware of Frerichs's brain studies. *Haberling-Hübotter-Viererdt Biographisches Lexikon der Hervorrangenden Ärtze* (Gurlt et al. 1930: vol. 2, 613–14) has a comparatively long entry on Frerichs but does not list "Über Hirnsclerose" among the long list of citations, nor does it include any mention of his brain pathology studies among his medical accomplishments. Later German compendia of medical history maintain this pattern. Even Colin Lee Talley, who pays more than usual attention to German MS research, depends on Charcot to say that "Frerich [*sic*] of Breslau" mixed a number of cases that were not *sclérose en plaques* in among his descriptions of cases that were thought to be (Talley 1995:6). Frerichs then had become at best a counterexample to Charcot's efficiency.

Frerichs's student T. Valentiner (1856) continued the study of brain scleroses, expanding the number of cases and forming a list of symptoms associated with the pathology confirmed at autopsy in some of the cases. Of particular relevance to the history of multiple sclerosis were the onset of paralytic symptoms on one side of the body (hemiplegia), the changes in speaking and the precedence of motor over sensory disturbances. But Valentiner studied the pathology of brain and spinal sclerosis in and of itself and did not distinguish among different kinds of sclerosis, either as tissue changes or in the living patients' symptoms. He was especially prone to include cases of mental illness among the nervous diseases and to assume that the presence of the same symptoms must imply the existence of scleroses whether or not there is an autopsy to confirm that. He automatically grouped with brain sclerosis an "idiot" paralyzed on both sides of the body. In this, his work was consistent with that of his predecessors in brain pathology, who associated mental deficiency during life with a "hardening of the brain" observable postmortem.

With the work of Frerichs and Valentiner, the tradition of finding brain hardening behind mental and moral defects entered the incipient study of MS. MS history is haunted by a diagnosis of brain sclerosis based strictly on symptoms but implying both a textural state of the brain tissue and a moral judgment on the sufferer. This in turn gave impetus to the attempt to distinguish diffuse sclerosis from disseminated sclerosis (MS).

Naturphilosophie, whether examining the makeup of the crust of the earth or stages of animal development, sought the elements of natural objects. Tissue had been shown to be made up of characteristic cells, and the gray lesions had been shown to be characteristic of one type of nerve tissue. Therefore, looking closely at the lesions might show the special cellular appearance of the pathology. Surface scanning of tissue did not provide the necessary level of comparison. Only the microscope could penetrate to the next level of focus. This might reveal what composed the lesions and how they had come about from normal tissue.

The first studies of cells were of normal cells as they formed visible tissues and of their normal development and function in organisms. Visible tissues were composed of collections of cells joined in various ways. But diseased tissue revealed a cell structure and individual cells that deviated from the known normal forms.

Rudolf Virchow's doctrine of "one cell only from another," of great general significance in biology, was announced in his *Cellular Pathology* (1858) because it had peculiar import for understanding the cellular nature of tissue disease appearances. Nothing new was created in a diseased tissue; every degenerate cell originated in a healthy cell. Therefore, the disease process could be understood as the changes that one cell type underwent to become another. In tissue pathology doctrines like those of M. F. X. Bichat or of Carswell, the diseased tissue was a thing in itself that had come about as the result of humoral shifts in the previous tissue. Virchow did not accept that a given disease was specific to the sufferer: universal cellular processes were at work. Inflammation, with its visible tissue changes, was at base the result of an irritating stimulus that caused the cells to change and proliferate.

Virchow identified a substance that "prevails most extensively in the animal body." After examining a number of tissues chemically, he concluded that this substance was found in all tissues rich in cells but that "it is only in the nerve-fibre that we observe the peculiarity, that the substance separates as such." Elsewhere it is set free only when the contents undergo a chemical change or are subjected to the action of chemical reagents. Virchow used the name "medullary matter" (Markstoff) or "myeline" (from the Greek word for "marrow") for this substance (Virchow 1971:270–71). He then explained its role in the cellular pathology of the nerves:

> If the nutrition of a nerve suffer disturbance, this substance diminishes in quantity and indeed may under certain circumstances totally disappear, so that a white nerve may be again reduced to the condition of a gray or gelatinous one. This constitutes *grey atrophy*, or *gelatinous degeneration*, in which the nerve-fibre in itself continues to exist, and only the peculiar accumulation of medullary matter continues to be affected. [Virchow points out that the nerve deprived of its myeline continues to function electrically.] The axis-cylinder would therefore seem to be the real *electrical substance* of the natural philosophers, ...and the medullary sheath rather serves as an isolating mass, which confines the electricity in the nerve itself.

Virchow does not mention the sclerotic patches, but he does explain the nature of the "gray degeneration" in the white matter of the brain and spine: it is a loss of the distinct local form of this universal cellular substance "myeline" and a consequent diminution, but not loss, of nerve activity. In keeping with Theodor Schwann's cellular doctrine, he also suggests a "loss of nutrition" as the cause of demyelination: the myelin no longer has access to a continuous blood supply and so it starves.

The "electrical substance" that Virchow associates with the axon cylinder was the subject of experiments by the "natural philosophers" Johannes Müller of Berlin University and his successor Emil Du Bois-Reymond. Drawing on Carlo Matteuci's (1844) theory that electricity flows through the nerves, Du Bois-Reymond used storage batteries to demonstrate the specific nerve stimulations of electrical flow and conceived of particles of electricity specific to the nerves with a distinct shape and polarity, the "electrical substance." Du Bois-Reymond and his colleagues believed that there are many different kinds of electricity. Michael Faraday had in 1831 demonstrated electromagnetic induction before the British Royal Society and proved that all forms of electricity are the same, but it was a time before his techniques and views were accepted. Virchow speculated that myelin served as the insulation to keep the electrical substance from leaking out into the surrounding tissues.

Another of Müller's assistants, Robert Remak, provided the anatomical basis for this speculation. Remak had only an unpaid assistant lectureship without subsidy and had to conduct his experiments on the side as he practiced medicine. In studies based on the embryology of frogs, he disputed Theodor Schwann's free formation of cells and argued for a succession of cells by a process of division. He observed a fatty substance, which he called "medullary matter," lining some nerve axons but not others. Remak established an anatomical structure for the transmission of the nerve electricity that Du Bois-Reymond was attempting to trace. This work was the basis of Virchow's account of the electrical transmissions in the nerves.

Though the universality of myelin was contested by later investigators and its role in nerve impulse transmission was revised, Virchow's gray degeneration linked a tissue appearance in cerebral disease with a cellular pathology, the disappearance of myelin which led to disturbances in electrical transmission. It also suggested a vascular (blood supply) theory of MS that would be debated, tested and elaborated for the next one hundred years. Macroscopic tissue appearances had become microscopic cell changes.

The cells themselves were ever more visible during these years thanks to improvements in microscope design (brighter, clearer fields) and the use of stains developed as dyes by the German chemical industry. These dyes had originated in attempts to make artificial quinine from aniline, and eventually they would return to medicinal use as the first antibiotics. Though the practice of viewing fresh, dried or frozen samples had its tenacious advocates, the desire for a vision of the living cell led to trying to view cells with their fluids and internal features intact. Virchow and other microscopists cut tissue specimens into sections, delacerated (stretched) them and treated them with chromic acid or ammonia to harden them, eliminating some features and creating others. In 1858 Joseph von Gerlach recommended using carmine dye to make living tissue (*lebende Gewebe*) more finely visible under the microscope without causing damage. The dye colored the long fibers and bodies, though it tended to render some of their internal structures indistinct. From the 1850s to the end of the century, anatomists and pathologists in Britain, Germany, France and Italy were experimenting with and inventing stains to bring out specific features of tissue.

In the late 1860s Carl Weigert discovered that bacteria were present in stained thin (microtomal) sections of tissue from the lesions of all too readily available smallpox victims. Bacteria had been seen among other microorganisms for some time, but this was the first time they were identified in inflamed tissue. Weigert did not attribute the inflammation to the bacteria (which was just as well, since smallpox turned out to be primarily viral). He did use his observations to establish cell death as the beginning of inflammation, in opposition to Virchow's idea of an increase in activity, an "irritating stimulus" that preceded inflammation. The smallpox observations suggested that cell proliferation followed necrosis, hence the increase of fluids at the site. Weigert's findings centered attention on the dead cells in a lesion. Weigert was in the habit of exclaiming "Schiwa!" (in reference to the Hindu destroyer god Shiva) when he looked at diseased tissue under the microscope. This account of lesions impelled the pathology of MS lesions toward a search for the locus of primary cell death and the cause of that process. Virchow's irritation and Weigert's Shiva led to two dogmatically separate lines of research.

Weigert taught his younger cousin Paul Ehrlich how to use stains to see bacteria. Robert Koch had already demonstrated that bacteria do have a role in initiating wound sepsis. By finding a potentially infinite variety of specific agents behind disease, these bacteriologists promoted an account of disease at odds with the set types of cellular pathology. The same inflammation might be caused by different bacteria; the same bacteria might cause inflammation, atrophy, abscess separately or together. In Weigert's own work and that of his successors, there was a potential reconciliation between pathology and bacteriology. For the time, however, bacteria posed a threat to the still-under-construction edifice of cellular pathology types. Efforts to fit bacteria in or reject them entirely fill the study of lesions in Germany and England in the latter decades of the century.

The cellular pathology of nerve disease and even the study of the normal state of nerves were made more difficult by the irregular appearances of nerve tissue under the microscope. The smooth, striated structure of muscle or the pieced structure of squamous tissue had no analogue in the tangled fibers and fatty strings, the cells without nuclei and the nodes without walls that were being disclosed in nerve fibers.

After the Englishman A. V. Waller provided a powerful technique (1850–52) for the study of living nerve-connections, nerve cutting research with animals made it apparent that all the nerve fibers of the brain and spine were extensions of cells rather than special fibers or hollow tubes. The central nervous system was increasingly understood as an interconnected whole, though it remained a serious issue just how continuous the connections were on the cellular level. To what degree were local pathologies independent of the system; how were they the consequences of systemic pathologies?

In 1863 E. Rindfleisch focused on the areas of gray degeneration in the white matter of nerves with the understanding that they constituted cellular blockages in the operation of nerves. At the center of the sclerotic patch in a tissue specimen taken from a multiple sclerosis victim, he found a greatly dilated blood vessel with thickened walls. The myelin had been lost from the nerve sheath and showed some decomposition products, though the axon remained intact and the glia, a support matrix, had increased in number. This showed that an inflammation of the blood vessel came first, followed by the destruction of the myelin (gray degeneration) and the proliferation of the glia. The hardening of the lesion seemed to Rindfleisch the aftermath of the blood vessel changes and the destruction of the myelin sheath.

Rindfleisch was one of several researchers working out the roles of the cellular components of the cerebral and spinal white matter in the formation of gray degenerations of myelin. Valentiner, Türk, Virchow and other predecessors had introduced several of these components and suggested their relations. Different researchers drew up and emphasized different components in their studies because they used stains and preparation techniques that emphasized these components. The cellular pathology of each component might have a distinctive appearance in multiple sclerosis or it might be ambiguous, sharing its multiple sclerosis quality with other diseases. Most of the researchers were practicing physicians, and they drew their human specimens from patients whose histories they knew. Variation in microscopic appearances might be associated with the specifics of a case. There was a tendency, especially in the German studies, to seek universal pathological appearances and spell out biological variations without paying attention to the case history of the source patient. Animal specimens, showing the same cells as did humans, were especially convenient for study.

Virchow already knew that the nerve axons were little affected in the gray degeneration; they were subject to their own type of sclerotic decay (amyotrophic lateral sclerosis). Myelin was recognized only as a local deposit of a common binding substance (the same substance that makes the hen's egg such a delight in the kitchen, Virchow wrote). Charles Robin and Louis Ranvier, with the aid of myelin-specific stains discovered during the 1860s, were tracing its unique configuration on nerve sheathing and were beginning to show that it was more than an insulator.

Rindfleisch scarcely mentions myelin in his analysis of the lesions. He concentrates on the blood vessels supplying the nerves and their pathology. Blood vessel degeneration initiates pathological changes in the nerves, as it does in other body tissues. Rindfleisch does recognize that the fibers generally classed as glia increase in number and infiltrate the site of the lesion. Virchow had named them "neuroglia" in the belief that they formed a neutral "glue" holding together the active nerve tissue. Weigert's development of a glia-specific stain (1885) showed that the glia have a cellular nature (nucleus and wall). The notion that an infection of the glia (gliosis) might be involved in multiple sclerosis became established.

Assessing the priority of these components in the pathological process was one aim of research. By the time he published the sixth edition of his basic text (*Lehrbuch der Pathologie*) in 1886, Rindfleisch was still convinced that multiple sclerosis was primarily vascular in pathology (that the initial cell death took place in the blood vessel), but he needed to fend off those who believed that the nerve fibers, the glia or some other element was the prime focus of MS.

The role of these components was being asserted on the basis of microscopic evidence verbally described or depicted in line drawings. The use of oil-immersion lenses and more intense artificial lighting improved the microscopic image and the quality of photographs, but there was no means of reproducing these photographs in print (through offset) until the last decade of the century. Those reproductions were so grainy that they could not show crucial individual cells. As late as 1919, a histology article (Klingman 1919) included drawings of cells but had photographs of stained tissues. Attempts to assert one description or another of lesion formation depended on words and drawings during the early years of MS cellular pathology.

This language and the controversies it organized really originated in the work of the Germans of divergent interests — from Marx to Rindfleisch and the succeeding generations. Whereas Marx was isolated and his work largely unknown, Frerichs, Valentiner and Virchow formed schools and disseminated their techniques, their quests and their quarrels through their students. For decades Virchow edited the main German-language medical journal, *Archiv für Pathologische Anatomie und Histologie und für Klinische Medizin*, usually referred to simply as *Virchows Archiv*. This came to include articles that ranged over all the learned domains — including archaeology, linguistics and natural history — but the journal was especially devoted to reporting new research in pathology and its clinical dimensions. In an 1876 article, the clinic of Nikolaus Friedreich (1876:120–28) compared multiple sclerosis with "paralysis agitans," commenting extensively on the diagnostics of Jean-Martin Charcot, a Parisian neurologist whose definitive clinical studies were gaining international notice.

5

An MS Milieu

When the Prussian army assaulted Paris in 1871, Jean Cruveilhier's former student Jean-Martin Charcot remained at the Salpêtrière, the old hospital for mentally ill women. Here, from his own clinic, he wrote to his family that he could hear the cannons of the invading Prussians pounding the city (Goetz 1987:155). This is more than a historical highlight: whatever went on in the outside world — wars, panics, springtime — it seemed that Charcot and his followers were enclosed in their wards with patients and specimens, barely listening to the outside. At the same time, Charcot successfully cultivated the political patronage and international prestige he needed to continue his research and teaching.

Originally a gunpowder works, the Salpêtrière was first a prison and then a depot for insane women, who were chained to the walls of its large cells. It was at the Salpêtrière and its counterpart for men, the Bicêtre, that the late-eighteenth-century physician Philippe Pinel ordered that the insane be distinguished from criminals and released from their chains, though they still were to be imprisoned.

After his academic medical training in the rigorous French national program, Charcot was assigned to an assistantship at the Salpêtrière (1848, another revolutionary year outside). This unenviable posting was probably the result of his working-class origins. Later, when he had an opportunity to request an internship site, he chose the Salpêtrière once more. There he remained the rest of his life, developing his studies, eventually being given his own clinic and laboratory, assembling a large staff of students and colleagues and holding his dramatic demonstrations of illness and healing for Paris society.

Charcot chose the Salpêtrière for reasons analogous to Charles Darwin's decision to travel as the captain's companion on a cramped survey ship: access to study materials. Even as an apprentice physician, Charcot recognized the variety of illnesses that had been deposited in the wards and the opportunities for investigation they afforded. As a hospital resident, he could examine newly arrived cases and follow their histories.

Those in the Salpêtrière's wards were considered incurable. They could only be used as tools to understand the nature of their afflictions. The Salpêtrière was like a natural history museum, with living specimens to be identified and compared with each other in life and in death. But the specimens seem to have learned how to make lives for themselves as well.

In 1861–62 Charcot and Edmé Vulpian authored a literature review on *sclérose en plaques* and paralysis agitans (Parkinson's); they adduced only one clinical case of sclérose, from another clinic (Charcot and Vulpian 1862). The sources cited were almost entirely German: little clinical and no histological study had been made of the diseases in France since Cruveilhier's atlas was completed in 1842.

Charcot set about rectifying this omission. With interns and students in his clinic, he sought to define the sclerotic lesions anatomically. In a set of lectures first presented in 1868–71 and repeated with modifications until their printing in the first volume of his collected works, edited by Bourneville and other former students (1892), he gave a precise clinical account of the disease. This *sclérose en plaques* is the collective product of Charcot's clinic, with some disagreements still expressed. A careful analysis of the researches of Duchenne, Vulpian, Ordenstein, Bourneville, Marie and many others shows rich variety of experience and opinion continually being reduced to the dogma of Charcot's clinic and training. In his "lessons," he repeatedly addresses those others as an audience of "Messieurs." For their part, they fill in the footnotes with theses and articles commenting on Charcot's main observations.

Sclérose en plaques occupies the sixth through the ninth lessons of the first volume of Charcot's collected works, right after paralysis agitans. In his brief history of research he gives Cruveilhier credit for first mention; he notes that while *sclérose en plaques* was almost completely forgotten in France, German physiologists beginning with Ludwig Türk, made it a subject of study. Recognizing the need to resume research in France, in 1862 he and Vulpian gathered examples that Bouchard, a senior colleague, presented at a medical congress in Lyon.

The macroscopic anatomy of the lesions is Charcot's first interest. His own drawings of specimens were the basis of plates reproduced in an appendix to the book and exhibited during his lectures. At the beginning of the lecture, he uses the images to review the exterior distribution of lesions, on the brain, medulla, spine and peripheral nerves. This wide distribution of plaques no doubt gives the disease its quality of seeming like so many other nervous diseases.

Turning attention to microscopic anatomy, he acknowledges that the histology of nerve tissue is new and contains many questions still under debate.

Just describing the lesions means voicing an opinion in this debate. To make matters simpler, he concentrates on spinal lesions, but he does not confine himself to the fibers and the cells and their associations in the white or gray nervous matter. He will focus attention on the connective medium (*gangue conjonctive*) of the spinal cord defined by Cruveilhier in his medical dictionary of 1820. He adds later that this is what Virchow called "neuroglia" and Kölliker "the reticulum." This tissue has a primary role in pathological changes in the central nervous system and especially in *sclérose en plaques*.

Charcot then reviews the appearance of a spinal section treated with chromic acid to make it receptive to carmine stain. The plate he refers to in this section comes from the German histologist Deiters and shows in color the features brought out by the stain. At the center of each nerve section, surrounded by myelin, like a small globule, is the red-colored axon. These sections aren't contiguous but are separated by a lightly stained substance that seems to fill all the spaces between the nerves. This is the gangue conjonctive, or neuroglia, which contributes significant mass to the organ. Within this mass are visible — at this weak magnification — ramifying enclosures that yield branches that themselves branch, crossing and recrossing to form a net with irregular openings ("*mailles*"). This structure becomes particularly evident in those places where there are no nerves. A more thorough examination of both lateral and lengthwise stained spinal sections shows that at points, the net forms nodes (myelocites or neuroglial knots) that seem to be the centers from which the branches of the neuroglia emerge. This network is visible in preparations of spinal section with chromic acid, which tends to exaggerate the fibrous nature. Some critics have said that the network is an artifact of the preparation and is not real. Fresh sections without acid, however, also show the neuroglial network; the acid preparation seems to bring about changes like those in the earlier stages of MS.

Having reviewed the normal tissue, Charcot is prepared to consider the pathology of *sclérose en plaques*. These results are a compendium of his and Vulpian's researches and of the work of Valentiner, Rindfleisch, Zenker and Frommann. He has been especially influenced by Frommann's book devoted to the histological analysis of a single section of the spine. The study is based on both transverse and longitudinal sections hardened in chromic acid and colored by an ammonium solution of carmine dye.

The spinal sections showing lesions exhibit concentric rings of progressive tissue transformation. On the periphery the branches of glia have thickened, and the nodes are enlarged and have multiplied in number. Moving into the transition zone, the nerve fibers have become thinner, and several of them seem to have disappeared due to the loss of their myelin. Now the branches of the glia have been replaced by thin threads like those found in ordinary conjunctive tissue, arranged parallel to the axon cylinders. They have become so reduced in volume that they hardly are visible in a cross section. They have invaded the gaps left by the loss of myelin, thus effacing the netlike aspect characteristic of the neuroglia.

At the center of the lesion all trace of the net has vanished, both the branches and the cells, and the nodes are fewer and smaller than on the periphery. They are visible here and there forming small groups in the spaces among the thin threads of the branches, which now fill completely the areas left by the disappearance of the myelin. The axons persist, mixed in with the threads but lacking the great size they have in the outer zones. They might even be mistaken for newly formed threads. This transformation of neuroglial branches into thin threads is peculiar to *sclérose en plaques*. It is not observable, at least not to this degree, in other gray degenerations of the white matter, for instance in locomotor ataxia.

After reviewing the same degeneration in longitudinal section, Charcot turns to the question of the threads. Are they the remains of the neuroglia, or are they a preexisting matter exposed and transformed by the degenerative events? Charcot cannot say for sure, but his information favors the neuroglial source, supporting Frommann's thesis. He passes quickly over the changes in the blood vessels, thus signaling his rejection of Rindfleisch's vascular hypothesis. He spends much more time on the globules and granules found in the mass of the lesion. As Virchow did, Charcot identifies these as the products of the breakdown of the myelin (he illustrates them in a drawing similar to that in Virchow's text). The gray matter suffers a yellow degeneration caused by the cells of the neuroglia themselves undergoing a concentric degeneration.

Charcot asks what condition of the neuroglia leads off the pathological process that ends in a transformation into *sclérose en plaques* but not into other scleroses of the central nervous system and infections of myelin. Drawing on the German tradition stemming from Virchow, Charcot shows that the answer comes down to an investigation of what makes the changes in the neuroglia different in pathologies that lead to the formation of plaques. Further research continuing in France and Germany followed the lines that Charcot emphasized. Histological research on MS was a study of the interplay of glial inflammation, myelin degeneration, vascular changes and alterations of the axon.

Pathological anatomy was only the introductory lesson to Charcot's *sclérose en plaques*. The Germans concentrated on their samples beneath microscopes. Charcot had a clinic with patients he could follow from admission to autopsy. Reviving Cruveilhier's clinical pathology, Charcot equated brain and spine degenerations with observable symptoms.

After pointing out that there are three basic anatomical distributions of the multiple lesions — cephalic, spinal and mixed or cerebro-spinal — Charcot chooses to concentrate on the mixed form ("the most interesting and frequently encountered form"). To set the theme for his approach to the nosology of mixed MS, he recounts an anecdote (Charcot 1892: vol. 1, 222–23):

A highly distinguished doctor, but one as yet unfamiliar with the symptomatology of MS (sclérose en plaques) came to visit one of my colleagues at his clinic. To show him professional courtesy, my colleague presented this doctor with a new illness: a fine specimen of the cerebrospinal form. Leaving his bed, the patient took several steps into the room. "An ataxic," declared the visitor. "Perhaps," responded my colleague, "but what do you make of the rhythmic movements shaking the head and upper limbs?" "It's obvious. It's chorea or paralysis agitans." The patient was then questioned. He answered with a very marked difficulty pronouncing the words, scanning his syllables in a special way, and often with a light trembling of the lips preceding each word. "Now I understand," the doctor returned, "you've tried to shame me by presenting me with a most complex case. Now there are symptoms typical of general paralysis [a euphemism for neurosyphilis]. Let's not go any further. Your patient brings together in himself the whole of nervous pathology."

This vignette of colleague and doctor-patient relations exposits Charcot's primary clinical issue of MS: it resembles several other conditions. It was a story repeatedly told in European and American clinics to initiate students and outsiders into the mysteries of MS; for instance, it was stated almost verbatim in a lecture by Joseph Hirschfelder (1882) at the Medical College of the Pacific in Palo Alto, California.

Charcot's exploration of the symptomatology of MS consists in the first place of telling the disease apart from other conditions it strongly resembles. In these lectures Charcot instructs his students in the secrets of differential diagnostics.

Like the authors of the pathological atlases, he gives the professional-in-training clearly discernible signs that will allow one to identify and predict the course of an individual's affliction. He is remedying the technical inadequacy of the earlier works. Since the time of the atlases, and in Charcot's own maturing experience, the specific links between pathology and symptoms have been ever more clearly defined. Rather than looking at the spine and brain and trying to guess effects of departures from the normal, Charcot defines behavioral signs (*caractères*), knowing their general location, which he can then elaborate on. The entire sixth lesson is dedicated to the histology of MS lesions. The lithographs of lesions themselves, the former center of pathological anatomy, are relegated to an appendix, and the drama of symptomatic distinctions takes center stage.

Charcot's exposition of mixed MS symptoms in the seventh lesson proceeds by distinguishing MS from the other trembling and paralytic conditions with which it is frequently mistaken. In effect he restructures the anecdote of the visiting professor, showing how to separate genuine MS from each of the other disorders.

The difference between MS and paralysis agitans (Parkinson's) is in the volitional initiation of MS tremors. An MS subject will tremble only when he or she attempts to perform an action and only in those limbs performing the action. A Parkinson's subject trembles all the time and throughout the body, ceasing only with rest. The other clinical points of distinction between Parkinson's and MS appear only after the patient is observed through the course of a history; the contrast in trembling is immediately diagnostic. Citing published papers by his student Bourneville, Charcot gives examples of the intentional trembling of MS: a hand shakes as it raises a drinking glass to the lips; the lips shiver before and after a word is pronounced. In an earlier lesson (number five) on Parkinson's, he points out that the distinction in tremor types actually goes back as far as Galen but that his instances introduce a considerable refinement.

The histology of Parkinson's is different from that of MS — its specific pathology had not been identified — but that is not visible to the examiner who needs to determine the condition from what he sees in the movements of the patient. Parkinson's may have been identified well before MS, but now it was being used to define MS by opposition of type.

Another characteristic contrast between MS and another condition was the arc of motor performance. In chorea, a tremor named for its resemblance to a dance movement, an action once commenced could be broken or halted completely (*"troublée, dès l'origine, par des mouvements contradictoires"*), whereas in MS, an action, shaken as it is, is usually completed (*"persiste en dépit des obstacles occasionés par les secousses du tremblement"*). And progressive locomotor ataxia is known by the erratic rhythm of the involuntary movements, as opposed to the orderly and sequential quality of MS movements. "You will see how, in the very moment of grasping an object, the fingers stretch out and extend excessively toward the back of the hand. Then the object is taken all at once almost convulsively with a sudden and disproportionate motion of all the fingers. This is only true of ataxia; you will never observe anything like it in sclérose en plaques" (Charcot 1892: vol. 1, 231). Using a patient to demonstrate the locomotor ataxia contrast, Charcot points out that ataxia symptoms can be found mixed in with MS when the lesions occupy certain portions of the spinal column posterior. Here Charcot refers to Cruveilhier's patient Paget, described earlier, whose inability to hold a sewing needle without a visual aid Charcot associates with the extent of her lesions on the upper posterior of the column. Cruveilhier did not draw this specific clinical anatomical equation. With his greater experience, Charcot is fulfilling the potential of Cruveilhier's reported material. Paget's MS is a specific kind of MS.

These three contrasts — Parkinson's, chorea and ataxia — give a kinesic figure of MS. They are like stage directions for a performance of the MS body. Charcot also recorded the pattern of tremors by attaching the hand of a patient to a device that activated a pen inscribing a horizontally moving roll of paper: each type of tremor had a different signature. The still photography that Charcot used to document the stance and expressions of patients was not adequate to describe the distinguishing tremor types. Charcot had to rely on other means to convey the difference.

He advises, however, that these motions in MS are not visible in any limbs while the patient is at rest and that they tend to disappear in time, especially with the growing feebleness of the later stages of the disease. It is important "to question carefully patients in whom this [trembling] symptom seems to be lacking."

Charcot considers trembling a symptomatology of spinal MS. Cephalic MS has its own set of symptoms: problems with eyesight, speech and thinking. Location of lesions generally dictates the type of symptoms, making it possible at least to predict from a patient's behavior where the plaques will appear when brain and spine are laid open to view.

Amblyopia, one of the most lasting of the symptoms of cerebro-spinal MS, offers a primary insight into the functional effects of the lesions. In people complaining of a simple weakening of vision among other MS symptoms, autopsies show that the lesions may occupy the full thickness of the optic nerves. This demonstrates that the lesions do not cut off the nerve function, though the nerves "in the trajectory through the sclerotic plaques, may be stripped of their myelin coating and reduced to axonic cylinders" (Charcot 1892: vol. 1, 234). Though Charcot's own idea of what the nerves actually do was unclear, he could detect the oddly integral nature of the MS lesion, which altered the visual appearance of the nerve entirely but did not impede its function. Nystagmus, the wandering eye symptom he considers next, is a more pronounced clinical sign of MS but does not offer such a dramatic instance of the nature of the lesions.

Still more common than the visual symptoms is what Charcot refers to as "*un embarras particulier de la parole*."

> Speech is slow, drawn out and at times almost unintelligible. The tongue seems to be "too thick" and at times can even recall drunkards speaking. A careful study can lead to the discovery that words are as if scanned: there is a pause between each syllable, and they are pronounced slowly. There is hesitation in speaking the words, though nothing that might be called a stammer. Certain consonants — l's, p's and g's — are particularly difficult to pronounce.

There is no degeneration of tongue or throat muscles, as in paralysis; however, the gradual loss of the ability to speak can strongly resemble the course of a general progressive paralysis. As in paralysis too, speech is often preceded by a nearly convulsive contraction of the lips. There can also be difficulties in swallowing and breathing in the latter stages of MS and progressive paralysis.

The advent of this mixed form of the disease, which Charcot refers to as cerebro-spinal sclerosis and as multiple sclerosis (*sclérose multiloculaire*), is often marked by feelings of vertigo. Patients describe it as a sense that objects in the vicinity are spinning around at a great speed: it can be sustained even with the eyes closed. It renders the walk tipsy. Though chronic diplopia can have the same effect, that ceases with the eyes closed. This continual vertigo distinguishes *sclérose multiloculaire* diagnostically from locomotor ataxia and Parkinson's disease.

Most of those afflicted look a certain way. "Their attention is vague and uncertain; their lips gape and remain half-open; their facial features show weariness, sometimes even a stupor.... What seems to prevail in these patients is a nearly stupid indifference with regard to everything." They break out laughing or start crying for no reason at all.

Charcot saves for last a discussion of the effects of the disease on the lower members of the body. The legs and thighs, usually one before the other, weaken and seem heavy. The foot turns out of the way walking, and the entire leg bends under the weight of the body. Usually, however, the slow progress of the paresis (partial paralysis) allows the patients to continue moving about. They may have to toss the leg forward as they walk. Eventually they reach the stage of having to stay in bed. They have an impression that their legs are growing massive or being prickled. Yet the skin retains its sensation and the muscles much of their tone. Here Charcot refers to "faradic" stimulation — applying an electrical shock to the muscles of patients — which demonstrates that however weakened, they have not lost their electrical contraction (*contractilité electrique*).

Throughout the symptomatology, Charcot refers to the manifestations by his patient Mademoiselle V. Now he gives a detailed description of her state on March 24, 1867 (three years prior to the lesson). Mlle. V's lower member paresis was so pronounced that she could walk only with the help of two aides. While walking, she threw her feet forward ("as ataxics do"). When she closed her eyes, she swayed so strongly that she would have fallen if not supported. She had lost tactile sensation in her lower limbs, and she could not describe the position of her limbs while her eyes were closed. She sometimes had sudden, sharp waves of a burning sensation (*violentes crises de douleurs fulgurantes*), and she felt a painful constriction about her waist ("like a belt," recalling Paget once more, whose case Bourneville refers to in his note: Charcot 1892: vol. 1, 244 n. 1).

Charcot reminds his audience that these are symptoms of locomotor ataxia. While they were predominant, this — rather than MS — might have seemed to be the diagnosis. Occasionally ataxia symptoms, together with a few of those symptoms characteristic of MS (tremors in the extremities, losing speech, vertigo and nystagmus), form a mixture itself more diagnostic of MS than the usual MS symptoms alone.

Charcot does not believe that this appearance of ataxia symptoms in MS patients is the result of the simultaneous presence of both ataxia and MS pathologies on the spinal column. He has never seen this in a cadaver but does not doubt it is possible. In most cases, the combination of symptoms seems to be due to the invasion of plaques into the area usually afflicted by ataxia's softening. In his note, Bourneville cites several cases traced from symptoms to autopsy.

Beyond this combination, Charcot adds instances of muscular atrophy. He also gives a portrait of the "spinal epilepsy" (described by C. E. Brown-Séquard) of MS patients, in which the legs contract on themselves entirely, with knees locked together, and exhibit contagious trembling upon stimulation. This is the "tonic" form of MS, distinct from the "saltatory" form suffered in ataxia and other spinal diseases.

His exemplary patient Mlle. V did eventually display tonic epilepsy, but she had not shown this by the time the lectures were given in 1870. The apoplectiform (stroke-like) attacks that often present themselves over the course of the disease and often end the life of the patient (*terminent la scène*) had not occurred. This is not to say, he adds, that these attacks won't begin for Mlle. V as well some day.

In keeping with Cruveilhier's example, and those provided by the Germans, Charcot was most comfortable expounding the spinal form of MS and to some extent the cerebro-spinal forms. He shied away from a detailed consideration of MS only of the brain.

The apoplectiform seizures he takes up at the beginning of the eighth lesson are not peculiar to MS, again illustrating how the disease may exhibit symptoms and even pathologies associated with other diseases. When considering the variety of seizures that often ended the lives of patients, seizures that bear a resemblance one type to the other, he was generally unable to locate anatomically in the brain and spine more recent lesions that could explain the sudden violence of an attack. Only old abscesses, lesions and cavities were present when the brain was opened to view, implying that the final progress of the disease was the outcome of their long-term effect and not of a suddenly appearing "congestion" as some have theorized. Measuring changes in the temperature of the brain can distinguish diagnostically between true apoplexy (abrupt stroke) and "congestive" (slowly building) attacks, which have similar external symptoms but different brain effects.

Another dimension of Charcot's work tracing the evolution of MS in typical cases is how the succession of symptoms through time can facilitate diagnosis.

> I have proposed to establish three periods in the progressive development of the disease: the first extends from the appearance of the first symptoms to the point at which the rigid spasticity of limbs reduces the patient

to virtual immobility. The second includes the period, yet longer still, during which the patient, restricted to bed or able to take a few steps in the bedroom, hardly is able to maintain life functions. The third begins at the moment when, as all the disease symptoms worsen simultaneously, the nutritive functions palpably diminish. This is the time with respect to the final period, to bring up the accidents which in the normal course of things, mark the end of the disease and lead to the loss of life.

Often the brain symptoms — vertigo, diplopia, speech failure and nystagmus — mark the first period. Intention tremor and limb paresis are likely to join these sooner or later: together, they enable a strong diagnosis. Spinal symptoms — weakness and partial paralysis of a lower member, often lasting over months or years and showing a tendency to worsen and extend to an upper member — are yet more common. And they make the situation of the clinician very difficult. A hundred years after Charcot's formulation, the *Merck Manual* was (and is) listing the same symptoms and signs and issuing the same warning against mistaking for MS symptoms that might indicate a curable disease. Recall Cruveilhier's lament at Paget's death due to pleurisy, which he mistook for an effect of her spinal disorder.

The partial paralysis that signals the advent of MS is also typical of a number of other afflictions; however, several other, lesser symptoms might be present to point out the true diagnosis. That MS is not initially accompanied by loss of sensation, atrophy of muscle or incontinence/retention should also help separate it from different paralytic disorders. Complete remissions sometimes take place during the first phase of the disease, holding open the promise of a complete cure some day. But they offer only vague information about the disease. The very outset of the disease is also sometimes signaled by gastric crises, which include cramps and heavy, repeated vomiting, but gastric symptoms never mix with the usual ensemble during the main course of the disease.

The initial symptoms — paralyses and visual degeneration — intensify as the disease advances, leading to muscle contractions and, in the last phase, loss of appetite, diarrhea and general wasting, incontinence, loss of intelligence and the abrupt advent of "bulbar paralysis" (where the medulla oblongata has been affected) — inability to swallow and, finally, to breathe.

In the rare cerebral and the more common spinal forms of MS, the lesions are confined to these areas, but the symptoms are not limited. The most common form is cerebro-spinal, which usually goes through its entire cycle in about six years. The spinal form can take a lot longer, up to 20 years.

Charcot is much less prolix on the causes of MS, which he confesses are completely unknown. He refers to Rindfleisch's vascular hypothesis. Conceding that the blood vessels do degenerate along with the nervous reticulum, he does not accept that the vessels succumb first and cause the nerves to follow suit. According to his observations, the pathological changes in both proceed at the same pace without influencing each other. But Charcot's testimony was not decisive in ending the career of the vascular theory.

The anatomical location of the plaques (*ilots sclérosés*, Cruveilhier's phrase) does seem to correspond to some external symptoms. The loss of motor coordination, the loss of position sense and burning sensations can be correlated with the invasion of the posterior portions of the spinal column up to a certain height. On the other hand the usual development of plaques on the front and side portions of the spinal column appears to be related to complete paralysis or paresis of the limbs and the rigid contraction of the muscles. Nystagmus and loss of speech appear in accord with plaques on the broader section of the brain stem. And there are the throat and lung muscle symptoms classified as "bulbar" or relating to the medulla oblongata.

Other symptoms are difficult to localize. In general, however, Charcot maintains that the axons, deprived of their myelin coating in the midst of the lesions, must transmit voluntary impulses irregularly, causing the shaking that troubles the performance of intentional movements. This axonic disruption isn't unique to MS, but it manifests itself in these lesions more than in other scleroses of the central nervous system. This may be why paretic symptoms progress so slowly in MS: the nerve transmission is slowly disrupted rather than completely blocked by this particular kind of lesion.

Charcot states that little is known of the conditions favoring the development of MS except that women are more likely than men to be afflicted. Adding 16 new cases to the 18 already reported by Bourneville and Guérard, Charcot cites a total of 34: 9 men and 25 women. The same collection of cases shows that this is a disease of youth or of the first part of adult life. It is found in 14-, 15- and 17-year-old subjects, usually occurs between the ages of 20 and 25, and rarely appears first after the age of 40.

Charcot can cite only one example in which MS seems to be hereditary. There are vague indications that repeated migraines or neuralgias predict the later onset of MS. Prolonged exposure to a cold, humid environment seems to have precipitated a number of cases. That factor was among the few also mentioned by Carswell in his case and by Cruveilhier: it seems to be a survival of an older humoral diagnosis of nerve trouble stemming from an excess of cold, humid phlegm.

> But patients most frequently invoke circumstances of the moral order to explain their illness. Prolonged stress [*chagrins prolongés*], for example those among others occasioned by an illegitimate pregnancy, or the conflict and unhappiness [*les désagréments et les ennuis*] accompanying a more or less false position in society, as is often the case with the institutionalized. This is true of women. The men mostly are social failures [*gens déclassés*], outside the mainstream, highly impressionable and ill-equipped to carry on what is called, in Darwin's theory, the struggle for

60   MULTIPLE SCLEROSIS

the preservation of life (*Struggle for life*). That commonplace etiology lies at the base, so to speak, of all chronic diseases of the central nervous system.

After his extensive examination of symptoms and anatomy, Charcot finally visualizes his patients as social beings responding pathologically to the emotional and social pressures of their lives. Like all other sufferers from nervous disease, these people have failed to situate themselves strongly and honestly in the social world: they lack the "nerve," as we would put it in contemporary English, though the French of Charcot's day did not have that expression. Charcot evokes Charles Darwin, but his women and men are subject to the same forces as are characters in the naturalist novels of Émile Zola and Gustave Flaubert.

Prognosis takes up an even shorter paragraph. "Will it always be the same?" There is some hope that physicians one day will learn to take advantage of the remissions that take place in a large number of cases and prolong the remissions into a cure. For the present, Charcot notes, we must remember that the disease becomes known only when the lesions are very deep and beyond the reach of curative means. Charcot thus tied any hope of healing MS to early diagnosis, which had to be achieved by knowing signs and symptoms.

After saying this, Charcot adds, "Would it be right for me to spend much time on therapy?" (*Irai-je, après ce qui précède, vous entretenir longuement de thérapeutique?*) He lists several commonly used antispasmodics: gold chloride and zinc phosphate only exacerbate the symptoms; strychnine relaxes them temporarily, as does silver nitrate, which has the disadvantage of worsening the spastic contraction and spinal epilepsy. Hydrotherapy brought a passing improvement in one case but not in another. Arsenic, belladonna, ergotic wheat and potassium bromide were all found to be worthless. He would say the same of electric shock and continuous current electrotherapy but advises more experimentation.

With this brief excursion into failed symptomatic treatment, Charcot concludes his lessons on multiple sclerosis. He mentions the disease several times in the other lessons of his complete works, mostly to compare the symptomatology and pathology with those of other conditions of the central nervous system, most notably Parkinson's disease and amyotrophic lateral sclerosis. During the years he delivered these lessons, Charcot and his students published a number of papers and theses on specific aspects of MS and other diseases, for instance on the thermometry of the brain and on the use of electrotherapy.

The three lessons on MS occupy only part of the first volume of the six thick volumes of Charcot's collected works. Charcot had his own industry and vigor to contrast with the quivering weakness of his patients: his vision of those suffering from lung disease, for instance, is not so categorically dispraiseful. Even as he seeks to define MS down to the very signs of its detection, he cautions on the ease of mistaking it for the effects of syphilis, Parkinson's and other diseases themselves not so well defined. MS recurs repeatedly in the other books of the works as a standard or a symptom mass to be excluded on the way to distinguishing a particular illness.

Charcot uses four phrases to designate the affliction: *sclérose en plaques*, *sclérose en ilots*, *sclérose multiloculaire* and *sclérose disséminée*. The first two refer to the appearance of the lesions, and the second two refer to the distribution of the lesions. They all distinguish MS from the variety of other central nervous system tissue pathologies that were identified and being identified in Charcot's time. *Sclérose en plaques* was Charcot's preferred phrase, and it became the key phrase for his students and for French discourse about the disease. There are no English or German phrases that easily correspond to it. Spanish and Italian physicians, whose languages can accommodate such a formation, did occasionally use a similar phrase. The small hard patches seemed to define the disruptive paralytic progress of the disease as well as suggest the mystery of its slowness and incomplete effect.

Sclérose multiloculaire, which probably comes from the German *multiple Sklerose* or the English "multiple sclerosis," identifies the number of different cerebral and spinal places affected by the disease and thus the mixed variety of symptoms shown. It distinguishes the pathology from the specifically localized or broadly generalized hardening of other scleroses. There are numerous hardenings. *Sclérose disséminée*, which becomes "disseminated sclerosis" in English, refers to the seedlike scattering of the lesions (though they don't always look that way). The multiplicity rather than the specific character of the lesions is again the concept presented.

It might be argued that *sclérose en plaques* is most precise because the *plaques* is plural and the *sclérose* conveys the multiplicity as well as its nature; but "multiple sclerosis" conveys the lack of precision that Charcot himself expressed. In carrying the aims of pathological anatomy forward into clinical pathology, Charcot was elaborating a disease that itself contradicted those aims. The pathology of MS was known, could be studied on the tissue itself and under the microscope and was readily distinguishable from other lesions, and the symptoms were so well recognized that they could be grouped in phases. Yet as Charcot illustrates with his anecdote of the visiting colleague, MS in the living patient could look like any one of a number of other clinically well-defined diseases. For Charcot's generation of physicians, MS had become the mystery within the precision created by their own method, much as syphilis had been for previous generations. And the two always seemed to mingle.

An astute clinical observer like Charcot must have longed for a means of opening a living patient's skull and spine to learn if lesions were present. This is a trajectory for the future development of medical imaging technology: to be able to look into the living. Medical thermometry, which had been initiated by Georges Martine in the early eighteenth century and made into a science by Charcot's older contemporary C.R.A. Wunderlich, seemed to hold some promise of judging internal states through careful measuring of regions and changes in temperature. Charcot also believed that "faradic" stimulation (mag-neto-generated current as opposed to "galvanic" battery current) could be reveal-ing. But none of these methods could expose the type and distributions of lesions hidden beneath skin and bone. Only the equation formed by observing the patient and later seeing the autopsy, repeated again and again through many variants, could provide the basis for knowing what to expect inside a patient who presented a specific combination of tremors and visual disturbances.

Charcot became so confident of this ability to project internal states from external behavior that he could predict the succession of symptoms in indi-vidual patients and the existence of pathologies and linkages he had never actually seen. His confidence was in his own diagnostic ability and in a logic of disease. If there were hemiplegic symptoms in brain MS, then there must be paraplegic symptoms, though he had never seen them. It was only a mat-ter of time and research; what he couldn't accomplish himself would be left for his students. As Cruveilhier wrote at the end of his diagnosis, an exami-nation of the lesions themselves might hold a key, might point a way back to some symptom that would prove unfailingly diagnostic in a manner expected but not yet known.

Charcot also set his students on the task of investigating MS. Indeed, he commanded those with the greatest promise to carry forward his insights in the hope that this would lead to an explanatory break. The title of Joseph Babinski's thesis, *Étude anatomique et clinique sur la sclérose en plaques* (1885), exemplifies the continuation of the clinical-anatomical tradition from the early years of the century. Yet Babinski's eye is on the structure and pathogenesis of the lesions. He examines the absence of degenerations secondary to the plaques, which come about only when the axons, usually intact within the plaques, themselves are subject to a primary degeneration. He dismisses the theory that the loss of myelin is the result of mechanical pressure on the nerves by conjunctive tissue and says instead that it is the organic result of nutritive nerve and lymphatic cell activity. And he summarizes the histology of MS (Babinski 1934:312–14): "The nature of the degeneration of the nerves, as observed in the cross-section of a nerve ending, in the vicinity of the section, is the persistence of a large number of stripped axons, the considerable alter-ation of the vascular regions and the almost complete disappearance of myelin from the center of the sclerotic patches — these constitute the histological essence of sclérose en plaques." This summary, then, serves as the basis for yet-finer delving into cellular details: it is another surface to be penetrated, just as Babinski penetrated the one set by Charcot.

Babinski also pursues Charcot's research agenda by showing the histological similarity between tabetic sclerosis (neurosyphilitic spinal sclerosis) and MS and between destructive myelitis and MS. Thus it is possible to sort out one further type of MS — *sclérose en plaques à forme destructive* — in which the axons are destroyed as in myelitis. The variations in the disease become that much more understandable.

He also creates another, new subcategory to include those cases where there are MS symptoms but no lesions (*dont les lésions echappent complétement à nos moyens d'investigation*). The précis of symptoms has become so tightly defined that in a thesis prepared under Charcot's supervision, Babinski can declare there is a pseudo–*sclérose en plaques*, which lacks what was, since Cruveilhier, the one essential feature of the disease: its lesions of specific distribution and texture. In seeming to provide one more diagnostic tool, this new name confirms Charcot's formulation of MS as a definite category that varies as it is specified, like the motion pictures that were beginning to animate still photography.

Babinski went on to discover a simply assessed neurological sign that can show the presence of tabetic and other central nervous system damage but does not always respond to the presence of MS lesions. He continued Charcot's work of defining and categorizing MS, and like Charcot, he followed cases and made further observations on the disease throughout his career. For both, however, the disease was a problem better stated and not solved. Their aim was to enhance the physician's skill of diagnosis, but even that seemed an elusive goal.

As Charcot bequeathed confidence in MS diagnosis to his successors at the Salpêtrière, so he bequeathed uncertainty about the real nature of the disease and the need for a decisive sign at the center of that analysis. MS was not the dramatic illness he was seeking in order to show the physician's mastery of symptoms. MS slide samples or the slowly limping MS patients could not attract the field of society visitors who came to the shows of hysteria he staged at the clinic during the 1880s. MS, as he constructed it, was a slow, insidious disease that might come and go and could not be induced through hypnosis.

Goetz, Bonduelle and Gelfand (1995:113–19) treat Charcot's MS as a piece in the neurology he designed, dependent on anatomical-clinical analysis, case study through time and the search for decisively indicative diagnostic signs. In having done so, Charcot raised expectations that the same questions might be answered about MS that had been (or were being) answered about infectious diseases like syphilis and cholera: was it a primary disease condition or the result of another infection with a completely different set of causes?

Charcot defended his contemporary Louis Pasteur, a chemist and not a physician, against condemnation by the national medical body, but he did not adopt Pasteur's approach toward treating disease. Pasteur's bacterial and chemical understanding of infectious disease was centered around vaccine development. Charcot and his followers did not think of MS and other non-transmissible diseases as susceptible to vaccine treatment. Classification and categorization seemed more appropriate.

6

Cases

The first number of the British medical newsletter *The Lancet* reported the case of W. Hicks, a weaver, 44 years old and "of spare habit" (September 1, 1827: 701-2). Mr. Hicks came to the hospital complaining of a partial paralysis of his hands, numbness, dragging feet and vertigo, for which he was given medication and cupped. He returned not long afterward with partial loss of power in his hands, and though he had no pain, he was unable to move his eye outwards. In fact he had been squinting at his work for the last seven years. Dr. Elliotson, replacing Mr. Hicks's previous physician, diagnosed a disease of the brain and possibly a tumor. He prescribed that the weaver's head be shaved and a tincture of iodine be applied twice daily. There was no improvement in his legs, and the weakness in his hands increased with a tingling in his arms, but the vision in his right eye was better.

The *New York Times* on March 16, 1996 (p. 36), reported the sentencing to jail of a man, George Delury, who had assisted the suicide of his wife, Myrna Lebov, by giving her a cocktail of an antidepressant, water and honey. Ms. Lebov was chronically ill with MS, and in a note dated the day before her death she said that she had asked her husband to help her die. However, Mr. Delury kept on his computer a diary, which suggested that he "had been at least partly motivated by self-interest." Transcripts of these diary entries disclosed Mr. Delury's wish to be free of his wife's needful presence. He also admitted his intention to turn the diary into a book showing "the complex, tortured feelings associated with taking care of a loved one who is so ill." Confessing that he had violated the New York law against assisted suicide, Mr. Delury plea-bargained the second-degree manslaughter charge to a guilty plea to second-degree attempted manslaughter and was sentenced to six months in prison, of which he was expected to serve four months. His book was, indeed, published.

Between these two cases, 170 years apart, printed in different journals for

different audiences, lies the history of MS cases. Mr. Hicks, the weaver, had
an ailment with some few symptoms of MS. The thought that he might have
been afflicted with that rather than with a tumor or a form of "brain disease"
can come only to a post–Charcot reader. MS organizes information differently
in retrospect. The decisive details are forever missing, which begs the question of whether or not there can be diagnostically decisive details for MS. St.
Lidwina, Heine and d'Esté are also cases of this sort, and a great many more
can be unearthed from medical journals prior to the early 1860s.

Multiple sclerosis is in the subheadline in the article describing Mr.
Delury's plea-bargain. Here the focus is not on Ms. Lebov, the person living
with MS, but on her husband, who was judged guilty of a crime. After being
mentioned in the headline, MS is not described at all in the article. It is
assumed to be a chronically disabling, incurable disease. Mr. Delury's diary,
intended to be a book expressing his agony as primary caregiver, is unlikely
to illuminate MS itself.

In history, cases change from the obscurely medical to the obscurely jural
and the publicly confessory, all fraught with revelations of personal details.
The paralyzed limbs and the opened spine and brain come into view, are
divorced from any individual patient, turn into cells and finally are just chemical reactions and court proceedings. The medical case becomes a legal case
becomes an act of publicity for a book. The individual life and even the name
are lost; MS becomes the name, replacing the victim's name in the headline.
A hundred years will pass before MS victims (will there ever be a better designation? MS'ers?) assert their own identity in print.

Plain clinical-anatomical reportage of MS brought it to attention as a disease, and such cases remain the basis of a medical education. They are available in textbooks and in interactive form (MRI given, you diagnose) on the
Internet. From the first detailed clinical analysis of MS up to the codification
of Charcot's lecture series, the presentation of MS cases within the medical
profession (not for or by the general public) grew more complex. MS had to
bear an ever greater symbolic burden as it was prepared to become a disease
of some public significance, with the combination of catchall ambiguity and
implied scientific certainty that such diseases require. Watching the development of MS cases shows the variety of ways in which the disease was envisioned and understood within the life materials of its victims.

Charcot's first MS case became a professional legend because it typified
insight and dogged research into randomly encountered disorders, characteristics that the neurologist must cultivate. Though only sketchily reported in
Charcot's own writings, it became one of the hallmarks of Charcot's success
for the young Sigmund Freud, who described it in his eulogy to Charcot. This
was published in the Viennese counterpart of *The Lancet*, the *Wiener Medizinische Wochenschrift*, on Charcot's death in 1893 (Freud 1963:16).

During his student days chance brought him into contact with a charwoman who suffered from a peculiar form of tremor and could not get work because of her awkwardness. Charcot recognized her condition to be "choreiform paralysis," already described by Duchenne, the origin of which, however, nothing was known. In spite of her costing him a fortune in broken plates and platters, Charcot kept her for years in his service, and, when at last she died, could prove in the autopsy that "choreiform paralysis" was the clinical expression of multiple cerebrospinal sclerosis.

For Freud, Charcot's astuteness in recognizing an already described condition in a living person gave him the opportunity to trace the history of the disease from inception and uncover its nature in an autopsy. This was the classic case procedure, which, as G. B. Morgagni himself wrote, depended on the good fortune of the examining physician to be able to follow a case from life to death. Charcot added patience (and ambition) to his perspicacity. He was able to form his clinical case by engaging the woman in his domestic service, making it possible to observe her daily and keep her close over her remaining years. Where Ollivier d'Anger's patient vanished after his clinical interview, the charwoman "specimen" was dependent on Charcot for her livelihood and perhaps for what medical care she could receive.

The phrase "*le service de M. Charcot*" was ambiguous. It meant service both in his house, in whatever servant corps Charcot had the means to maintain, and in his clinic, to be under his care as well as at his command. Clinical cases developed within the service of a physician, and patients, if able, might be given tasks within the clinic or household of the attending doctor. By 1882–83, when the French government under Gambetta founded a chair of neuropathology in the Paris faculty of medicine for Charcot and expanded his clinic at the Salpêtrière, the service of M. Charcot had become a ramified and complex order, encompassing a number of clinicians, interns, students, workers and patients in varying relationships. Often the patients were, as cases, identified by the location and number of the bed occupied.

The unnamed charwoman was Charcot's act of self-identification in his profession, but Mademoiselle Josephine Vauth, often referred to as Mlle. V., was his lecture epitome of what he discovered. Her name appears to give Charcot's own example of, for instance, visual symptoms or apoplectiform attacks; he adds her to others cited throughout his lecture from the cases reported in the literature or by colleagues. Charcot's case notes in the Bibliothèque Charcot at the Salpêtrière are quite detailed and were the main reference for students to consult; Bourneville summarizes Mlle. Vauth's clinical pathology in a note to the eighth lesson (Charcot 1892: vol. 1, 264–65 n. 1).

Josephine Vauth is Charcot's case of the elementary form of the disease. The apparent initiation in the aftermath of (an illegitimate) pregnancy, lower-limb symptoms progressing to upper limbs, visual deficiencies and spasms and

finally death by asphyxiation together form the predicted course; only speech
symptoms go uninstanced here. The autopsy, which concentrates on the spine,
affirms the affect of lesion location and position on bodily capacities. The brain
lesions are mentioned but not detailed, though it is implied that they were
present in the medulla at least.

Against this collection of disease elements, Charcot juxtaposed what he
called *cas frustes*, that is, cases that differ from the typical. *Cas frustes* open the
possibility of matching symptomatic differences with pathological differences
and build a picture of the disease itself. After he set down the histories of,
and could exhibit patients with, the core of typical symptoms, Charcot sought
the deviations, to study and also to exhibit.

An example of a *cas fruste* of *sclérose en plaques* that Charcot placed before
his audience in December 1876 was that of M.-A. Fisch, a woman 24 years
old at that time (Charcot 1892: vol. 1, 423–24).

> At the age of 8 she experiences severe pain and was unable to move her
> lower limbs. She was confined to bed for six months. When she started
> to walk again her right foot was lame. Seven months later lameness of
> the left lower leg forced her to stay in bed for several months. In 1873,
> while at the Salpêtrière, she has a series of *epileptiform attacks*, foaming
> at the mouth. Later her upper limbs become lame and one notes a
> difficulty of speech, her sight grows weaker; when the patient laughs her
> mouth remains half-open. Over the course of the next year, one observes
> a worsening in the parts of the lower limbs seized with a spontaneous
> shaking and, in a moment, there follows a trembling of the right hand
> as voluntary movements begin. In 1874 the symptoms are the same except
> that the speech difficulty is more pronounced [pun in both French and
> English]. Today (December, 1876) the following symptoms are present:
> rigidity of lower limbs when extended; spontaneous and evoked shak-
> ing; rigidity and paresis of the upper limbs, especially in the right one;
> absence of any trembling in voluntary movement. Sensation is not
> impaired. Speech is a little hesitant, but, in this at least there is an
> improvement over the state two years ago. No trembling of the head or
> nystagmus. In a word, this patient shows marked improvement in cephalic
> symptoms.

Charcot had divided MS into cerebral, spinal and cerebro-spinal types, each
with its typical suite of symptoms and course of development. This, however,
is a departure from the usual development of spinal symptoms in not com-
pleting the course, a *cas fruste* in the most positive sense of possibly providing a key to the healing of the disease. *Cas frustes* are, by their very nature,
unlike each other; the typical pattern remains typical to be violated by the
unusual ones, whether of spontaneous remission, sudden severity or unusual
symptoms.

This notion of case histories goes beyond the illustrative to the dramatic. Charcot exhibited his patients in his lectures, juxtaposing the normally ill with the deviants. These exhibitions were the most publicly visible aspect of *le service de M. Charcot*. They earned him a reputation outside the confines of the specialty he and his students were creating. Freud was only one of many foreign students, specializing graduates and visiting dignitaries who came to hear Charcot's lectures and see the exemplary patients paraded before the audience. The nerve-afflicted were of course the most dramatic; in them the written cases came alive and offered the possibility of electrical and even surgical experiments. The hysterics, both men and women, became the great attraction of Charcot's shows, stimulating the development of one form of psychiatry but also contributing to a decline in Charcot's professional credibility. The turn to hysteria epitomized Charcot's later investment in a theater of illness. Making a public entertainment of cases is one of the less endearing heritages of neurology.

No one else had Charcot's institutional control over patients, his ability to follow them for long periods of time or his capacity to anatomize a body whose behavior he had long observed. His categories born of and in these facilities spread far and wide, but the ability to realize them as Charcot did scarcely ever accompanied their use.

With the publication of Charcot and Vulpian's researches in 1867–68, the clinical and the histological pattern of MS became available to practicing physicians. A thesis by Charcot's students Bourneville and Guérard (1869) commented upon the main points and was in turn reabsorbed into the growing edifice of Charcot's clinical lectures, from the start a collaborative work progressively published by Charcot and a number of others in French journals, especially the hospital gazette *La Lancette Française*. As early as 1870 the American physician Meredith Clymer was commenting on Charcot's discoveries and detecting MS cases of his own. In the mid–1870s, translations of Charcot's works began to appear in English, American and German journals, but well before that time, knowledge of his school's diagnostics and treatments had spread.

Though it was clear that Charcot's histology and even his cases at first derived from work outside of France, the model that Charcot provided was an extremely suggestive way of envisioning cases where the outward signs seemed unrelated to each other. Practitioners had seen enough of these specific symptoms together to welcome the authoritative catalogue and nomenclature developed in France. An experienced practitioner, Sir Samuel Wilks, could even write in 1873 that he and others had long been seeing the lesions but had not made anything of them. Charcot's diagnostics was differential, founded on distinguishing *sclérose en plaques* from Parkinson's and neurosyphilis varieties such as ataxia. That was sufficient to make it a diagnostic object.

Charcot's MS did not enjoy universal acceptance even within the closed world of French clinical medicine. The staged effectiveness of the clinical lectures, attended by colleagues from all over Europe and America, helped spread Charcot's particular "doctrine of the nerves" to other countries, where it was received, debated and adapted to local medical diagnostics and practice. MS in Charcot's formulation was one more element in a growing cosmopolitan medicine that, like other developments in Western science, was shared and debated across boundaries even as the countries themselves warred with each other. The Franco-Prussian War was a sound of cannons to Charcot; wars, insurrections and social turmoil reverberate in the forming edifice of MS.

Perhaps the rapid growth of American cities during the latter decades of the nineteenth century, the increase in the number of patients and the relative openness of the medical profession there made the United States a primary site for the spread of the MS case pattern. The daguerreotype, another French product (imported by Samuel F. B. Morse, 1839), was already enjoying in America a prosperity that it had never found elsewhere, not even in France. Americans were not just passive recipients of European medical knowledge, though European training was considered an accomplishment and a recommendation. Surgical anesthesia had been pioneered in the United States, and several new forms of surgery, some of them unfortunate, had been introduced there. American medical journals, hospital gazettes and newsletters, like their counterparts in Europe, described cases that only needed Charcot's paradigm to be considered multiple sclerosis.

One of the earliest physicians outside France to attempt to assimilate Charcot's work into his practice was Meredith Clymer, the New York specialist in nervous diseases (he never referred to himself as a "neurologist"). Clymer states: "To Dr. Charcot unquestionably belongs the credit of distinguishing this condition [disseminated sclerosis] from other paralytic disorders and notably from paralysis agitans, and recognizing its pathologic features, and tracing its clinical history" (Clymer 1870:72 quoted by Goetz, Bonduelle and Gelfand 1995:119). He added: "[Charcot] has done for it what Chomel and Louis did for typhoid fever when they established it as a distinct species of continued fever, characterized by a definite group of symptoms" (Clymer 1870:231, quoted by Talley 1995:12). These words are from a series of three articles that Clymer published in New York state medical journals in 1870, full of his excitement after visiting Charcot's clinic and hearing the master's lectures.

Clymer's praise of Charcot was cited by a colleague, William Hammond, Professor of Diseases of the Mind and Nervous System and of Clinical Medicine in the Bellevue Hospital Medical College. Hammond had practiced as an army surgeon at various forts in the American Southwest, was promoted to general, was court-martialed for insubordination, had the decision reversed by Congress and went on to a prolific career in New York. Hammond's citation is in the first American review article on MS, "Multiple Cerebral Sclerosis," published in the strongly case-oriented journal *American Practitioner* (Hammond 1871b:129–50). The paper was to be a chapter in Hammond's more general treatise on diseases of the nervous system.

At the outset, Hammond notes that multiple cerebral sclerosis has been only recently recognized as a distinct pathology associated with certain symptoms and that the symptoms have caused it to be confused with groups of diseases, paralysis agitans and others, similar in symptoms but different anatomically. Hammond takes up the cerebral form of the affliction because he is able to describe this from his own observations, using his own cases as illustrations.

Pain is the first symptom to appear, followed by tremor and then paresis in the affected limb. He does not find that the tremor is exclusively intentional; this may be true of cerebrospinal sclerosis but not of cerebral sclerosis. Without once referring to Charcot (or yet to Clymer), Hammond eliminates one major distinction between MS (all types) and paralysis agitans (Parkinson's). Inability to maintain contraction for a sustained period of time and thus to coordinate muscles generates an agitation independent of the underlying tremor, the results of which are observable in attempting to draw a straight line with a pen. This "loss of appreciation in the state of the muscles" has appeared under different names in the case literature, but Hammond is sure it is all multiple cerebral sclerosis.

The patient of this disorder loses a knowledge of the exact situation of the several parts of the body, evident in the inability to touch a specific place with the eyes closed. The body is inclined forward, head falling toward chest, trunk flexed at the pelvis, knees slightly bent, moving ahead not at a walk but at a jog-trot. He recounts the story of an elderly man who had to be carried downstairs but who, once he reached the door, "went at a full run and jumped into his carriage without the least difficulty." This attribute of Hammond's multiple cerebral sclerosis sounds more like Parkinson's paralysis agitans than Charcot's MS [Parkinson 1817: "The propensity to lean forward becomes invincible. ... In some cases, it is found necessary to substitute running for walking, ... The chin is now almost immovably bent down upon the sternum"]. Also unlike Charcot's MS, Hammond's sclerosis is evidenced by tactile sensibility that is impaired from the start, and again, it is mainly a disease of the elderly rather than of the relatively young, as Charcot would have it.

Hammond's first citation of Clymer (1870:7) is of Clymer's doubt that multiple cerebral sclerosis is even an independent affliction. But Hammond is certain that it is; not only that, the "head-symptoms" (festination, alterations of sensibility, incoordination, muscular anesthesia) are "sufficient to diagnosticate multiple cerebral sclerosis from functional paralysis agitans, which is never a very serious affection." Hammond later returns to paralysis agitans and cites Clymer's opinion (no source given) that (excluding the tremor, which is secondary to the disease) there are two varieties of paralysis agitans, "first, that which results from multiple (disseminated) sclerosis, affecting the encephalon and spinal cord; second, a purely functional disorder, first fully described by Parkinson." In a note he indicates that he has not been able to obtain a copy of Parkinson's original treatise. The functional disorder has a tremor that shows no disposition to spread, has no lesion and is readily cured. The other "paralysis agitans" is actually Hammond's multiple cerebral sclerosis, which other authors have confused with multiple cerebrospinal sclerosis or considered an aggravated form of the functional disorder. Hammond, with the help of Clymer, thus shows that his multiple cerebral sclerosis can absorb Parkinson's disease, which is no longer to be assessed in a patient on the basis of the tremor.

Here Hammond presents the one case (of nine) he followed all the way to autopsy. "P. B., male, aged 65, formerly a drummer in the army, and latterly an instructor of buglers, came under my observation at Ceboleta, New Mexico, in the winter of 1849–50. While milking a cow, one evening, he suddenly experienced a severe pain in his head, which lasted only a few seconds. He soon afterward had an epileptic paroxysm, during which he bit his tongue severely." Soon thereafter, P. B. developed in his left hand a tremor that extended upward to his arm; then his foot began to shake, with subsequent involvement of the entire leg. The right arm and leg also acquired the tremor, but only the left hand and ultimately the left arm lost sensation. Before the tremor came to either leg, his body was inclined forward, but once both legs were affected he walked with difficulty but could impel himself forward at a trot. The tremor was continual during his waking hours and finally all the time, and this sleeplessness, combined with the poor nutrition of the barren winter on the western frontier, contributed to his loss of strength. His mental powers deteriorated from the first attack, and by the time he died, two years and a month after the first epileptic fit, he was in "a condition of very decided imbecility."

Hammond wrote that he made the postmortem without preconceived notions, but he did expect to find lesions of some sort. Opening the skull, he found the meninges healthy, and even after removing the brain from the skull and examining the base, he found no lesions at all on the base. Removing the meninges, he cut through the right hemisphere with the scalpel and encountered a spot of resistance. This turned out to be a mass of dense tissue; a thorough examination of both hemispheres turned up a number of similar masses of varying sizes (cherry stone to walnut), but there were none in any of the other encephalic masses and, despite a careful sectioning, none in the spine. Continuing with the food metaphors, Hammond found the textures of the "sclerosed bodies…, many of them, as dense and hard as cartilage, others were like hard-boiled white of egg, and others like cheese." He did not examine any of the tissue under a microscope.

This case, 20 years earlier, apparently fixed in Hammond's mind the pattern of multiple cerebral sclerosis, and he proceeded to diagnose others that came his way according to the symptom-pathology pattern he had identified there. He turned to treatment he most favors for the disease: simultaneous administration of chloride of barium and hyoscyamus (henbane, Hyoscyamus niger, a Dioscorean remedy for sleep disorders abandoned from pharmacy and then restored during the early nineteenth century as a treatment for epilepsy and nervous excitement). Hammond tells of a U.S. senator who came to him in 1870 with what had been diagnosed as "shaking-palsy" [Parkinson's] but what Hammond determined was actually multiple cerebral sclerosis. After one day of treatment with barium chloride and henbane, the senator began to improve, and that improvement continued, though the senator still took his medicines "and will probably be obliged to do so for a long time yet." Hammond also recommends electricity as treatment for multiple cerebral sclerosis: "I am not sure that it makes any difference in which direction the current be passed, but it is important that it should not be so intense as to cause any considerable pain."

Hammond had done research of his own to discover antecedent diagnoses of what had to be multiple cerebral sclerosis under other names, from Stoehr's hemispheres corpora mamillaria to Valentiner-Frerichs' cerebellar peduncles and Meynert's cerebellum and protuberance. None of them are a form of paralysis agitans, in which bodies of sclerosed tissue are found in the brain. In a fashion similar to Charcot, but without a clear knowledge of Charcot's clinical distinction between Parkinson's and MS, Hammond invented his multiple cerebral sclerosis from cases. Clymer may have proclaimed Charcot's distinction between MS (disseminated sclerosis) and Parkinson's (paralysis agitans), but his attempts to explain that distinction in the New York medical press crystallized Hammond's belief that he had discovered something with a sclerotic brain pathology and the symptoms of Parkinson's.

Readers of the *New York Medical Journal* would have known that Hammond had published, the month before (February 1871), another installment in his text on mental diseases, an article on "diffused cerebral sclerosis." Though he does not make the contrast in this or in his other articles, it would appear that he distinguished diffused sclerosis, which encompasses a large area of the cerebral hemispheres, from multiple sclerosis, which is formed of a number of separate patches. His studies of diffused sclerosis are based on secondhand material from other physicians, and even more than for multiple sclerosis, he extends the pattern to encompass cases that show what he considers crucial symptoms.

American medicine was still based on the experience of the individual physician, who made his own judgments and prescribed his own preferred remedies. The conjoint effort of an enclosed group of clinicians studying and treating a captive population of patients over time, as in Charcot's and other French establishments of that time, was not replicated in the United States, not even in the medical centers and asylums. Charcot's method of diagnosis did not influence older physicians, whose experiences were formed by a few defining cases of rare conditions. Even a transmitter of new doctrine like Clymer conveyed the ideas but not the method and social system that supported them, hence the doctrine lacked a local ground. Physicians were independent medical entrepreneurs who needed to promote their own doctrines, maintaining communication with each other by evoking common anatomical and pathological categories. Multiple cerebral sclerosis was the way a number of patients and medical students were going to know about certain kinds of mental disease until they began to receive their own cases. But for rare diseases like this one Hammond's 20 years and nine cases formed a persuasive precedent.

The degree and the quality of the penetration of Charcot's MS diagnostics into U.S. medicine are illustrated by another case (Noyes 1871), reported by one of Hammond's colleagues at Bellevue, Henry D. Noyes, who was Professor of Ophthalmology there. Miss A, a dressmaker of English birth, was brought to his office in September 1869 by another physician, who summarized her history of head and back pain and the loss of power in muscles of the mouth and tongue. Pain in the eyes, double vision and loss of sight, which meant loss of the ability to sew, were the reasons she came to Noyes. The double images were so far apart that they could not be corrected with prisms.

Miss A's eye muscles were subject to paresis and spasms. Using an ophthalmoscope (a narrow beam of bright light with a magnifier, invented by Hermann Helmholtz in 1851), Noyes discovered optic neuritis in both eyes, with infiltration into the optic disc but not the retina. He rendered a qualified diagnosis of brain tumor, but writing in retrospect, he noted that he regretted he had not paid much attention to the paresis of the ocular muscles and the tremor that established itself once she took to her bed after a severe visitation of headaches. "Her feet would jerk, and, as her sister described the effort, they would 'move on their own account.'" He prescribed potassium bromide, but with a tumor there was an unfavorable prognosis.

Noyes watched Miss A's symptoms worsen, her optic nerves atrophy, her vision degenerate and the strabismus and nystagmus appear. She had difficulties chewing and swallowing; taste and smell were impaired, but hearing was painfully intensified. Though Noyes does not describe her speech, he comments on the imperfect control of lips and tongue. The headaches were constant and sometimes produced partial spasms but never any convulsions. Her intellect was clear, and her secretion was more or less normal, but she seldom slept and slowly wasted away "through starvation and suffering. Her life flickered longer than I expected, and went out on the 30th of July 1871, without any new symptoms."

Because of the symptomatology, Noyes had explicit expectations of the autopsy, which two pathologists performed 24 hours after death. Though they had been informed of the brain symptoms, they could find no tumor or hemorrhage in what appeared to be a perfectly healthy brain. "The brain was incised in every direction; all the sections looked and felt healthy." There was no examination of the spine, nor was there microscopic inspection of any tissue.

"The unsatisfactory conclusion of this case gave me great disappointment. I was unable to account for its remarkable features despite the opportunity of an autopsy." Noyes' search of the literature brought him the "true explanation of the case in the hypothesis of disseminated sclerosis of the brain and spinal cord to which Charcot called attention." Noyes then refers to Clymer's 1870 articles in the *New York Medical Journal* and the *Medical Record*. He does not mention the *New York Medical Journal* articles written by Hammond, his colleague at Bellevue.

For Noyes, Miss A's symptom history, especially the "great and pathognomic symptom of tremor" conforms to the criteria Clymer presents from Charcot's work. Noyes is sure that a careful microscopic examination of the central nervous system tissue and the performance of chemical tests would have provided evidence of disseminated sclerosis, and he greatly regrets that they were not done while the specimens were available.

Three American physicians practicing in the same area, two in the same hospital, had three different diagnostic visions of MS: Clymer described Charcot's symptomatology of disseminated sclerosis; Hammond invented his own "multiple cerebral sclerosis," in part from Clymer's account; and Noyes realized that Charcot's disease as presented by Clymer would have been the best description of his case, had he known to collect the necessary pathological data. That these symptoms are beginning to be noticed and described together, and interpreted as a disease of nervous tissue rather than an intrusive growth or tumor, is a development mostly spurred by Charcot's own work. Hammond could read German as well as French, but neither he nor Noyes had the capacity to perform the kind of tissue studies that the Germans initiated and Charcot advanced. Charcot's and then Clymer's statement of a symptomatic package made vague nerve cases visible as emergent MS. Noyes' ophthalmological skill equipped him to associate optic neuritis, already a known condition, with disseminated sclerosis, though he did not have the cases to follow through on the connection.

It took a little more time, a fact remarked on by British historians of medicine, for Charcotian cases to appear in British hospitals. Almost immediately after the first publication of Charcot's results, German physicians were composing elegant case studies based on the clinical-pathological model provided (e.g. Schüle 1870), as well as continuing their own lines of histological and chemical inquiry. It was not until 1875 that "Two Cases of Insular Sclerosis of the Brain and Spinal Cord" was published in *The Lancet* (Moxon 1875b). The author of these cases, Walter Moxon, refers to them in the first paragraph as the "*sclérose en plaques*" of French authors.

Moxon published a longer study, encompassing eight cases, in *Guy's Hospital Reports* later that same year (Moxon 1875a).

> The recognition of this disease by English physicians will appear singularly slow at the time (which must soon come) when its characters are more generally known.
>
> Some disorders have received universal credit though they are only identified by symptoms without any certain morbid anatomy; such as paralysis agitans, &c. Other disorders are equally generally allowed, although they only have a constant morbid anatomy without any certain symptoms; such are cerebral abscess, &c.
>
> It must appear strange that the singular and definite disease of which I am about to relate a few cases has not yet been admitted by the profession in this country, when we know that it not only has constant and characteristic symptoms, but also a quite peculiar and very remarkable morbid anatomy.
>
> Although the two cases under my own care, of which I shall give the post-mortem appearances are, as far as I know, the only ones in which the diagnosis has been made sure by inspection after death, on this side of the channel, yet cases of insular sclerosis (sclérose en plaques, inselförmige sclerose) have been recognized and verified in France and Germany in many instances.

Moxon argues that although the disease certainly is polymorphous, its character is definitely established. Reflecting rather than following Charcot's procedure, he divides the "art of describing diseases" into the intensive and extensive directions, detailed description of the main symptoms and broad inclusion of all related symptoms. Favoring description of disease as the least number of characters that will establish a case, he lists the eight that decide a case as insular sclerosis. He then reviews each symptom in its normal expression and peculiarities. The object is to provide practicing physicians with a standard for detecting and describing these cases.

Moxon's formulation of intentional tremor leaves out the distinguishing intentional feature — he admits it is difficult to describe — and concentrates on the cessation of trembling when the parts are supported. He does not vacate the intentional category entirely, as Hammond did; he is sure this peculiar tremor is distinct from the other nervous oscillations, and he gives specific contrasts. But Charcot's deciding contrast is missing from this precise list. Moxon is sure that having once been seen, the tremor is so distinctive that it is unlikely to be mistaken afterward. In this and in other features, Moxon relies on clinical fellowship where verbal description fails: knowledgeable colleagues will point out the tremor.

The volitional element so important to Charcot is also absent from the speech symptom that Moxon says "attracts the attention of the careful observer at once. The words appear to cost too much pains, and to be produced one syllable at a time, each syllable accented, and yet not so distinct as a healthy person's accented speech." Moxon recognizes that this slow and distinct speech pattern does not arise from a paralytic affection of the tongue but may result from a small impediment or twitching action that causes hesitancy. It is not as if the speaker is trying to get a grasp of the whole of what he is saying and thus scans or counts out the words as he gives voice.

Tremor, paralytic weakness, absence of anesthesia, contractions and rigidity, nystagmus, little disturbance in power over excretion, normal electro-irritability, affection of speech and enfeeblement of mind are the eight symptoms Moxon holds as constant. The morbid anatomy of the disease is small hard patches distributed "indifferently" in the white matter of the central nervous system. How can this random distribution always produce the same basic symptoms? There are so many patches that "principle of average comes into play, and the symptoms are *a constant average result* of the numerous points of disease." Whether this means that so many lesions are always bound to disturb (or not) the functions that constitute the symptoms or that so many lesions always disorder the higher-level, integrated functions such as motion and speech, Moxon did not comment on. Hughlings Jackson and other contemporaries were beginning to find failure of integration in epilepsy, but Moxon did not pursue the implications of his neural averaging.

Moxon discusses the preparation and examination of tissue specimens and the pathological changes that can be observed in the vicinity of lesions. Because he did not maintain as strict a concept of localization as Charcot, he did not marvel at the persistence of function amid so much tissue damage, though he did notice how deeply into the sclerotic matter the axis cylinders in spinal matter retain their form while the other tissue is transformed. Like his predecessors, he could only infer the progression of morbid changes from the condition of postmortem specimens and conclude that normal features left unaffected by a general pathology must have some significance for the pathological process. He does not comment on the significance for the symptoms.

Like Charcot too, Moxon noticed that vessels often but not always appear at the center of sclerotic patches, but he did not suggest a vascular etiology of the inflammation preceding the hardening. After the model of the British pathological anatomy illustrated by Carswell, he seeks analogies between this sclerotic tissue and morbid changes in other organs, and he discovers in a form of ateritis changes that seem like sclerosis. But that analogy or another, a bone disease, cannot be useful, since the cause of the tissue damage is not known in either case. Moxon classes all these as "eruptive" diseases: "A local disease is set up by some agency which is of a specific kind, and is not native in the part in which the change is seen." This is a fresh insight into the nature of the MS lesion drawn from a tradition of pathology separate from Charcot's, an insight that, even if forgotten, can be repeated with the appropriate diagnostic training.

Moxon elicited the patients' own accounts of their health before the attack, which in each case was a visitation of weakness, often in the performance of work. Previous clinicians had made some note of history before admission. Moxon, despite his own rigid formulation of symptoms, took care to discover signs, what the people themselves thought had initiated or even caused their disease.

A common feature of the eight cases Moxon then describes in varying detail is a precipitating shock. The first case, a 25-year-old woman named Emily B. (a case that Moxon had already published in *The Lancet* in 1873), began to have symptoms after a febrile attack with diarrhea. She herself attributed her disease to finding her husband in bed with another woman. Another case was Matilda P. When a doctor, his hands covered with blood, emerged from the room where her sister was giving birth and announced that her sister had died, Matilda P. had a hysterical fit and a weakening of the legs.

Emily B., his earliest reported case and his model for the development of insular sclerosis, was an instance of both physical disease and psychological trauma. She confided to a nurse the story of finding her unfaithful husband. Her friends did not know about it, and only her evident trustworthiness in other areas gave the story credibility. She exhibited a "weakened" intellect, staccato speech, intention tremor and absence of other symptoms that might mark this as a different disease. "The jerky palsy of voluntary action of the limbs" specifies intention tremor better than Moxon's general description: you do need to see it in order to know it.

The postmortem gave the expected evidence of sclerotic patches in the white matter of brain; indeed, the entire brain was hardened and shrunken. Microscopic examination of the lesions confirmed the French and German accounts of histology and Moxon's own belief in the eruptive nature of the disease.

Matilda P. was initially diagnosed as a hysteric. Not long after admission and despite her appearance of health, she developed the suite of symptoms during life, her brain and spinal cord showing the grey patches of degeneration after death. The changes in her speech are in themselves diagnostic of her status as an early woman patient of insular sclerosis:

> ...her answers are sensible, and uttered in correct language, in a proper modest manner, but utterance is impeded slightly in a peculiar way, the accents dropping often on every syllable like a child reading a primer, or else falling on syllables that are not usually accented, while there is no distinctiveness corresponding to the accentuation. Sometimes several syllables run into one queerly accented sound; the general result being a syllabic sounding utterance quite peculiar, there being a want of that

conventional pronunciation in which we slur over certain syllables of words and bring others into prominence. She makes the wrong ones prominent, or all equally prominent.

The background of this description is the expected modulated speech of a young woman. The content of the speech is itself proper in both the grammatical and the socially correct sense, but the manner of articulation is hesitating and as if deliberate in each syllable. Moxon describes this same speech pattern for two of the men, but without commenting on the correctness of the language. One man speaks as if the words are being forced out of his mouth. In no case does Moxon describe the coprolalia that a few of Charcot's and Bourneville's patients produced. Most had sudden fits of laughter and crying.

Two of the patients died in the hospital, and their insular sclerosis was demonstrated in autopsy. The other six left the hospital in varying states of recovery; the only determination was symptomatic. The treatment was symptomatic, for tremor (silver nitrate, henbane and compounds), for constipation and for pain. The single treatment most frequently used was electricity: faradic stimulation and galvanic baths. This was directed at the muscles, to cause them to flex in response to the current when the patient had difficulty achieving that motion of itself. From the description of the treatment, there also seems to have been some expectation that it would help the nerves of the spinal cord and peripheral nerves.

Moxon states at the end of his article that the "results of the treatment used in the foregoing cases will be seen from the report to be most unsatisfactory; no approach to cure has been made." The patients may sound as if they are improving, but their record shows that they grow slowly and steadily worse. He lists the medications given, and like Charcot, he finds that they have no real power over the disease. Moxon also explains that his use of the phrase "insular sclerosis" instead of "disseminated sclerosis" distinguishes this disease from the other kinds of diffused disorder known as sclerosis, such as "miliary sclerosis," which had been recently described. Moxon detects the need for great precision in naming, since other disorders may be lurking within a too-general name.

Moxon's cases substantiate his general view of the eruptive nature of the insular sclerosis; they all have a sudden onset, and though those still living may leave the hospital after treatment, the prognosis is not good. The physician knows what will happen, and can do nothing about it. This diagnostic and prognostic knowledge, Moxon's cases also show, is becoming standardized among physicians. People of different genders, class backgrounds and manners of life can be diagnosed with the same kind of cerebrospinal damage. Charcot's teaching finds ground in cases that are used to educate other physicians and students (but apparently not patients) within an increasingly professionalized and specialized medical realm. As the common knowledge of insular or disseminated sclerosis grows, the elementary symptomatic forms are connected with the pathology, which is examined for causation. Variants are detected, named and classified. The history of MS goes forward in the formation of physicians' ability to recognize and classify.

The cases now reported in French, English and German medical journals are more likely to be the formes frustes of the disease, unusual variants of the known pattern that might illuminate its basis. As the variability of the pathology that can produce similar symptoms becomes clearer, a category of "sclerosis" arises, linking a general set of symptoms to conditions of central nervous system hardening. As was already evident in one of Moxon's cases, nervous disorders like hysteria can initially describe the behavior of patients who then can be judged sclerotic through a more specific symptomatic reading. Diagnostic categories like hysteria and sclerosis are vague until they are suddenly, dramatically specified in a case.

A case of "disseminated cerebral sclerosis" reported by the London surgeon W. Bevan Lewis in the "Clinical Notes and Cases" section of the *Journal of Mental Science* (Lewis 1878) shows the maturity of this method. The 33-year-old, "J.H.," a widower, was seriously depressed for about a year after the death of a favorite child. A week before he was admitted into the London West Riding Asylum, he became "restless, excited and eventually outrageous in conduct." The outbursts were "characterised by noisy incoherent raving and shouting, aggressive behavior, and dangerous and destructive propensities." This was reason to bring him to the asylum. The friends who brought him there did not give a consistent account of his history. It was clear that he had been leading a dissolute life and "lately had become very intemperate in his habits."

For the week after he was admitted, J.H. remained in a state of "acute delirious mania." He raved so violently, shouting profanities and nonsense, that his throat became dry. He moved about his room restlessly, not paying attention when addressed, his personal habits generally foul. "There was a profuse flow of saliva from his mouth." He received food only when it was forced into him with a funnel, and he had to be catheterized to release retained urine. He slept only under sedation. After a month of this behavior J.H. became torpid, apathetic and extremely feeble. He could no longer walk unsupported, his skin was cool, his pulse was a little fast, but he did eat food unaided. Then he took to his bed, lying motionless and not responding to questions. Developing symptoms of hypostatic pneumonia, he "sank" five weeks after admission.

The brain at autopsy showed considerable wasting over the lobes; the pia mater was tough, thick and congested. Beneath the thin layer of gray matter, the white matter showed a "distinct mottled congestion."

Microscopic examination revealed a condition of disseminated sclerosis of the white matter. The patches of sclerosis were very numerous and in constant connection with the vessels. There was abundant proliferation of the nuclei along the course of the vessels, and deposits of hemaetoidin crystals in the sheaths. The grey matter was unaffected, the nerve cells appeared normal, but the sclerosed patches extended up through the medullary strands as far as the spindle-cell or deepest layer of the cortex.

This case has none of the special symptoms that Charcot or Moxon associated with *sclérose en plaques* or insular sclerosis. Amid a condition of general cephalic wasting, the small sclerotic patches are distributed throughout the white matter of the cerebral cortex. Delirium leading up to apathy and a final paralysis are thus entered into the list of symptoms associated with brain sclera, and "sclerosis" moves one step closer to becoming a physico-mental condition like hysteria. Lewis simply reports the case as disseminated sclerosis on the basis of the pathology. The vascular alignment of the lesions seems to mark their origin: disseminated sclerosis is the primary cause of the other brain degeneration observed. No alternative cause, for instance alcoholism, need be given. The work of Charcot's student Gilles de la Tourette was not evoked. Spongiform encephalopathies (Creutzfeld-Jakob disease) were yet to be described.

Sclerotic pathologies were being interpreted to include secondary pathologies and a much wider range of symptoms to form a disease called disseminated sclerosis. Hammond and Lewis present cases with a strong focus on the physical fact, in the white matter, of many small sclerotic patches, which must cause whatever symptoms occur and must be present when these symptoms are present. They don't distinguish among possible textures of these patches. Moxon gives greater credence to a typical balance between certain symptoms and insular sclerosis. He makes a distinction between this and disseminated sclerosis, a uniform hardening, and miliary sclerosis, many tiny hardened patches. Lewis's case would be disseminated sclerosis in Moxon's sense, but it is not clear that Moxon distinguished any other types.

A paper presented by Edward Constant Seguin before the New York Neurological Society in February 1878 (Seguin 1878) summarizes the clinico-pathological state of the scleroses ten years after Charcot's papers appeared. The son of a Parisian psychiatrist driven out of his directorship of the Bicetre by the revolution of 1848, Seguin qualified at the New York College of Physicians and Surgeons before returning to study under Charcot in 1869–70. He was therefore quite familiar with Charcot's procedures and theories. In his paper Seguin discusses "disseminated cerebro-spinal sclerosis" in two described cases, with a detailed pathological anatomy of central nervous system tissue taken from both.

Seguin's first case, which was recorded by Dr. Van Derveer of Albany,

New York, was an unmarried 29-year-old accountant named Thomas Grogan. Grogan's mother and several brothers and sisters had died, though his father, a brother and a sister were still alive and in good health. Grogan was studious and fond of dancing until taken ill. His first signs were eye pain and difficulty sustaining the march in a military funeral. He had flashes of internal warmth, and any excitement made his flesh feel as if it were creeping. A pain in his ankle made him think he had sprained it when he knew he couldn't have. He and his physicians interpreted these episodes and the attendant weakness as the result of overwork, but the prescribed rest did not lead to recovery. He was troubled with "more or less flatulence, dizziness, loss of sight and constipation."

Feeling an improvement, Grogan went to a hot springs and took 100-degree-Fahrenheit sulfur baths, but that prostrated him. When he came under Van Derveer's observation, he had improved to the point of being able to walk unaided but unsteadily. He complained of serious weakness and a constriction around his body. His conversation was bright and fluent though he had difficulty pronouncing the two words "truly moral." As at the beginning of his illness he had spontaneous seminal emissions and eventually frequent erections and great sexual desire. He was given various medications to stabilize his nerves and help him sleep. Dr. Stevens examined his eyes with an ophthalmoscope and "diagnosticated sclerosis of the optic nerve." Seguin noted: "Dr. Clymer saw him about Oct. 1st, 1871, and observed the following more marked symptoms in his disease: Tone of voice drawling; brain seems weakened, and nystagmus of the eyeballs is apparent. Has, in addition, spinal epilepsy; it having only a general connection with sclerosis. The latter condition only occasionally present."

Grogan's "muscular will power" and his sensitivity to temperature and stimulation, especially on the left side, were impaired. "There is characteristic dragging of the feet, and the will power is inadequate to give the proper stimulus to the muscles, yet he displays considerable control over the leg when attempting to flex it." A treatment regimen of pills containing strychnine and ferric hydroxide did him no good. When Clymer saw him one year after his first visit, Grogan's muscular willpower was much weakened. He was wasting and showed symptoms of paralysis on the right side of his face. His sexual desires ceased. He had lost the ability to whistle, and as he approached death (February 21, 1874) it became difficult for him to talk. There was no aphasia, but the muscles of his mouth seemed to be paralyzed. There was no general postmortem; his brain and spinal cord were sent to Seguin for autopsy.

The second case was a single woman, age 23, with no name or hint of ethnic identity given. She was under Seguin's observation, a nervous girl given at times to hysterical laughter or tears. She began to feel weakness in her right leg after a long and vigorous walk and thought that she had sprained her knee. Her ability to use the leg fluctuated; sometimes she was almost cured, but she had finally come to require support. On examination, Seguin did find a paresis in the right leg and a lessened sensitivity to pain. "In view of the history of the case, the capricious development of the palsy, the absence of reliable signs of central disease, the presence of a strong neurotic element in the family, and the fact that strong emotions had been acting on her, I concluded that the patient had a functional palsy of an hysterical nature." A treatment of strychnine caused her to become tetanized, but with no apparent benefits afterward. As she became paraplegic and her hands grew paralyzed, she was placed in an "irregular water-cure house, she developed" where extensive bedsores developed. She soon died of exhaustion and pyremia. The postmortem showed disseminated sclerosis of the spinal cord.

Seguin performed an autopsy of the tissues from both cases. After a thorough topography of lesion distribution in the brain and the spinal cord of the first case and in only the spinal cord of the second, Seguin divided the morbid process of the histology into three phases. In addition to the granular dissolution of the myelin, Seguin observed in the neuroglia the growth of branching cells and the persistence of the axis cylinders of the neurons amid the degeneration. In the ganglion cells of the spinal cord there was a remarkable absence of these branching processes, with a few notable exceptions. Seguin found analogues to the branching cells in the reported histology of other nerve degenerations. There was nothing to associate these cells directly with the blood vessels. They appeared to be normal elements of the neuroglia that had hypertrophied. Again he could find comparable cell structures in the depictions of other histologists. The paper is followed by a page of drawings of the spinal cord sections, the preparation of which he carefully detailed, and drawings of the clustered protoplasm, the hypertrophied wall of the arteries and several of the branching cells.

Seguin does not attempt to align specific areas of brain or spinal cord degeneration with specific symptoms: his paper is innocent even of reference to bulbar symptoms or other well-recognized categories. He documents his cases as symptomatic disseminated sclerosis, makes a survey of lesion distribution then moves rapidly down to the microscopic realm of the cells. The tragedies of the dancing, whistling Irish-American accountant and of the nameless, hysterical young woman with her family history of disease are not directly equated with anything that went on within their central nervous systems. The same cellular pathology brought about the slightly similar illnesses and deaths of these two very different people. For there to be such consistent morbid changes in the same tissue — changes in existing tissue rather than the development of new tissue — there must be a consistent cause. Having made his histological observation and entered his evidence against the vascular theory, Seguin does not speculate further about causes. Cruveilhier's enjoinder to seek causes deeply in the pathological anatomy of the tissues continued to define research. But the most detailed account of the disease's pathogenesis does not give its cause.

This juxtaposition of individual cases with cellular pathology is unusual because pathology seeks general causes while case medicine looks to individual symptoms and cures. Seguin's paper illustrates the divide between these two approaches in the history of MS. He reported his cases to show that they both had the symptoms and that the same cellular pathology was at work.

Cases would continue to be reported abundantly over the next 30 years, but their only relationship to histology would be to make available tissue specimens of someone showing symptoms that deviate from those of the main of disseminated sclerosis. Symptom differences must be reflected in the tissues. Working under this assumption, physicians and anatomists had some surprises as the nineteenth century rode into the twentieth and as the library of cases grew.

7

Dissemination
and Differential

On September 20, 1888, the American neurologist Landon Carter Gray read a case history (Gray 1889) before the American Neurological Association. This told of an unnamed man, age not given, who had come under Gray's care at the New York Polyclinic. The man had chancre and papula irruption, symptoms of syphilis ten years earlier, but when Gray and his colleagues observed him he was showing "all the symptoms of a case of disseminated sclerosis." Gray even used the man as an illustration in his lectures at the Polyclinic. Intention tremor, nystagmus and scanning speech were continuous and apoplectoid attacks were repeated during the three years he was hospitalized. For six months before his death he was seriously demented and unable to care for himself, though he didn't weaken appreciably until right before death. Gray excluded other possible symptomatic explanations of the man's condition.

Twelve hours after the man's death, the autopsy disclosed a soft and edematous brain substance. A severe leptomeningitis, an infection of the pia and arachnoid maters, was spread all over the apex of the brain and the cerebrum, extending downward to the tempora-sphenoidal lobes and irregularly to the second temporal convolutions. "Careful search was made for sclerotic patches, but none was found; nor was there at any point the hyperaemia upon contact with oxygen of the air which has been so often observed in sclerotic patches." Further examination of cerebral areas and sections studied microscopically did not show any sclerotic patches.

Gray was able to locate one other similar case, leading him to conclude that "the tremor of disseminated sclerosis is due to lesion of the cortex or of the underlying white strands." He cites other cases of multiple and diffuse sclerosis in children, of paralysis agitans and even of experiments with cortical stimulation of monkeys to prove that it is any lesion of the cortex, not just

85

sclerotic plaques, that produces the tremor. The audience of neurologists whose remarks were quoted tended to agree that Gray's case indicated the patches did not have to be present for MS symptoms to appear. Dr. Mills went so far as to say that "some symptoms regarded as pathognomic were probably not due so much to the nature of the lesion as to its location in the cerebro-spinal axis." He added that disseminated sclerosis might also exist in the sensory tracts without showing a tremor.

As the assembled neurologists well knew, leptomeningitis pathology is often a central nervous system outcome of syphilis. The patient's earlier symptoms of infection (chancre and papula) made that a strong likelihood. If advanced neurosyphilis can mimic disseminated sclerosis so well, then symptomatology is not so good a key to the pathology in a patient showing typical symptoms. The diagnostic strength of Charcot's triad of intention tremor, nystagmus and scanning speech was thrown into doubt. The American Medical Association eulogy of Charcot (August 26, 1893) mentioned his work on locomotor ataxia, St. Vitus' dance and hysteria but not multiple or disseminated sclerosis. This was a change from Meredith Clymer's praises 23 years earlier.

E. Leyden's eulogy before the Berlin Society of Internal Medicine in 1893 did mention Charcot's study of *inselförmige Sclerose* and a number of other nervous conditions. For Leyden, Charcot's influence was too strong: German physicians were so taken with his descriptions that they felt obliged to go to Paris, sit for Charcot's lectures and come back to spread the doctrine in Germany. "The clinical method which is particular to our German school stresses much more in-depth analysis, careful research and critical examination of topics. Such qualities have been somewhat relegated to second place by the French school" (Leyden 1893, trans. in Goetz 1987:155). Sigmund Freud's eulogy, published in the Viennese medical newsletter, of course mentioned Charcot's *sclérose en plaques* in almost sentimental detail. But Freud was one of those German-speaking physicians who had gone to Paris and had brought back (some did and still do contend) the worst features of the late Charcot's studies of hysteria.

Hundreds of cases in 16 different languages (French, German, English, Russian, Spanish, Italian, Japanese, Portuguese, Dutch, Polish, Czech, Swedish, Danish, Norwegian, Romanian, and Hungarian) are listed in the second series of the *Index-Catalogue of the Library of the Surgeon-General's Office, United States Army* (1906). In addition to these, many more are accessible through national medical bibliographies, hospital records and physicians' records on deposit in libraries and other repositories. These cases collectively form an attempt to single out and label the disease. They also are a record of the spread of clinic-based case medicine from its European centers to secondary locations in Europe and the world outside. Disseminated sclerosis, in Charcot's and other forms, was becoming disseminated with the emergence of national medical institutions in many countries and with the development of a cosmopolitan medicine based on scientific Western medicine.

The Charcotian edifice was in the paradoxical state of being both the foundation that was used for recognizing *sclérose en plaques* and the barrier that had to be destroyed to permit clear-headed observation of new cases. Like a simple, highly persuasive religious tenet, the clinical properties of Charcot's disease gave a vision of symptoms yet permitted enough dissent and emendation to assimilate individual cases.

When, for instance, Dr. W. M. Butler of the Brooklyn Homoeopathic Hospital read a paper on disseminated sclerosis before the Kings County (New York) Homoeopathic Medical Society on December 10, 1889 (Butler 1890), he was careful to identify his case through the three characteristic symptoms. The case was a 22-year-old Norwegian builder who was brought to the hospital suffering from heat exhaustion; after two weeks in the hospital and treatment with oral medications and enemas, he began to show intention tremor, nystagmus and scanning speech. On the doctors' advice, he was sent back to Norway, presumably to be cared for by his own family.

Contrary to the tenets of their own medical theory, which they regularly violated in keeping with practical experience, the homeopaths had put the builder, who was showing a temperature of 108 degrees, directly into an ice pack on his arrival at the hospital. Their injections of brandy and administration of glonoin, beef-tea and whisky as his high temperature continued were more consistent: giving the chemically warm to the overheated. Butler believed that this was the first instance of disseminated sclerosis precipitated by sunstroke.

Variable as the etiology of disseminated sclerosis may be, its symptomatology, due to the different distribution of lesions in the brain and spinal cord, is even more widely variable. "Any description, therefore, of its symptomatology must be general and subject to multiple modifications in individual cases. No disease more emphatically emphasizes the importance of the revelations of that little army of quiet workers, who, by their experiments on the lower animals have revealed the peculiar functions of the different parts of the brain and the spinal cord. Only by the light of this knowledge could one understand how one and the same disease could present such varied manifestations." Though accepting Charcot's basic symptoms as characteristic, Butler opens the diagnosis (and implicitly the treatment) of disseminated sclerosis to great variation. He concludes the account reflecting Charcot's and many others' pessimism about a possible cure for disseminated sclerosis. Yet his assessment of the disease's protean clinical nature leaves open multiple possibilities for symptomatic treatment. His mention of "that little army of quiet workers" refers to the study of reflexes and localization that had continued from the work of Marshall Hall (*Memoirs on the Nervous System*, 1837) to his own day, using the experimental method to learn precisely which nerve location influences which bodily action in animals analogous to humans. No one had yet discovered in animals a disease like the MS they were studying in humans.

Maintaining a diagnostic standard for disseminated sclerosis led to a historical vision of the development of cases. Even where it was not possible to gather together a number of cases for comparative observation, a physician might glimpse a temporal relationship between cases. The most obvious relationship was familial.

Physicians routinely inquired into family background when taking down histories, to learn both if disseminated sclerosis was transmissible and if it was associated with any other conditions that had been passed from one generation to the next. Urban clinics, with their anonymous intake, were increasingly the locus of contact with patients showing a variety of conditions, but a great many physicians in European and American settings lived their entire lives in the same small town or rural center, were medical consultants to several generations of the same families and hence were able to note disease patterns. James Huntington described the condition that bears his name because he — and his father before him, also a physician — practiced in the same part of Long Island, New York, and saw the same families developing the same ultimately fatal disease generation after generation.

Alert to familial patterns, physicians concluded that familial disseminated sclerosis did occur but was so rare as not to constitute an etiology of the disease. The first comprehensive neurology textbook, William Gowers's *Manual of Diseases of the Nervous System* (1868: vol. 2, 544), announced that "direct heredity" (two or more siblings affected) was exceptional and that "indirect inheritance" (a general family history including forms of insanity, epilepsy or paralysis) was more common. At the beginning of his highly regarded account of disseminate(d) sclerosis in *Allbutt's System of Medicine* (1899: vol. 7, 51), J. S. Risien Russell concurred that more than one member of a family was rarely found to be affected. Reviewing these opinions in the context of his own research into the clustering of cases in two families, Dr. Ernest S. Reynolds of the Manchester (England) Workhouse Infirmary agreed that the disease is not often found in families, but he believed that "where one member of a family has typical disseminated sclerosis, another member who has been diagnosed to be merely 'neurotic' may really be found to be suffering from aberrant disseminated sclerosis" (Reynolds 1904:168). The opinion was seconded by discoveries of "suggestive" family history from Australia (Gill 1904).

The tendency of mental disorders, insanity, imbecility and hysteria to cluster in kin groups might yet disclose greater family inheritance of disseminated sclerosis. At the same time, disseminated sclerosis did seem to run in the company of a mixture of other mental disorders, what Drs. Irwin Neff and Theophil Klingman (1899:435) referred to as a "hereditary taint." In their examination of the family tree of one patient with "multiple cerebro-spinal sclerosis," Neff and Klingman found chronic nervous trouble, meningitis, hysteria, imbecility and epilepsy, as well as a number of deaths from consumption. For Neff and Klingman, the hereditary taint was a predisposition toward the immediate cause of multiple sclerosis in their case, which they believed to be "autointoxication from defective elimination," that is, the man became infected because he was constantly constipated in his youth. However, "the infectious process only joins hands with developmental or inherited tendencies; it may give rise to secondary disorders of cardiac, vascular, digestive or and metabolic origin." Their careful analysis of the cellular pathology of the case also showed an absence of marked changes in the vascular system, adding evidence against Rindfleisch's vascular theory of the origin of the lesions. They would have been interested in Charcot's observation that bowel disturbances often precede the emergence of *sclérose en plaques*.

Neff and Klingman's paper shows disseminated sclerosis in the process of becoming multiple sclerosis. On the one hand, it is a characteristic individual case with a specific and in this case "a special anatomical form"; on the other hand, it is the result of a family defect. Other infections present during the growth of the fetus may have had a bad influence on the developing central nervous system. Like many other physicians and biologists during these years when human embryology was becoming an active discipline under the guidance of animal studies, Neff and Klingman had difficulty separating hereditary causes from birth circumstances. Was the central nervous system of this one man affected because the family, and particularly the women, were diseased? (Childbirth was infection-ridden even for those not "tainted.") Or did the family heritage pass on a susceptibility to infection and an infectious etiology of mental disease?

The focus shifted from the individual case to the family and back to the individual case. The lack of strong evidence for a family transmission specifically of disseminated/multiple sclerosis tended to disqualify hereditary factors, driving explanation into vague, almost biblical estimations that could subsume all of the diseases endured by a family into a generality that covered their character and destiny. Neff and Klingman's patient had "physical stigmata of degeneration": his face was asymmetrical and prognathous; his body was covered with coarse and wiry hair; he was round-shouldered. Physical anthropology could then classify him with a larger class of degenerate humanity — criminals and the insane — whose physical attributes must include conditions like multiple sclerosis, whatever its immediate pathology. Where the family could not be the explanatory category, the anthropometric class did that duty. A look at the family disease chart of Neff and Klingman's patient shows that one of his many sisters died of marasmus, which is one way of writing "starvation." Anthropometric class seemed to have something to do with social class.

Infectious disease became the proximate cause of disseminated sclerosis, but family heritage and/or membership in a degenerate social order that probably influenced development became the ultimate cause. Questions of whether the disease was primary or secondary were moot when the disease became absorbed into the manifestations of human decay exhibited in hospitals for the insane and in public workhouses. Other family studies in New York (Mettler 1905) and Italy (Massalongo 1903) set a similar social frame for families afflicted with the disease.

By the end of the nineteenth century, disseminated or multiple sclerosis was still a rare disease of interest primarily to doctors and other treatment specialists. Connecting it with syphilis, insanity and imbecility made it unlikely to receive much publicity or acknowledgment from patients and their families. Though a few people left physicians' consulting rooms and clinics with a name for their partial paralysis and a regimen of treatments deemed appropriate, there was no mention of the disease in newspapers or other nonmedical public writings. It was not a stylish disease, like consumption (tuberculosis), nor was it a scourge, like cholera.

The number of reported individual cases grew in number and variety and were presented from outliers such as Mexico City (Gonzalez 1902) and Algiers (Scherb 1904) as diagnostic principles, European-trained personnel and texts spread from Europe. The European centers in which large numbers of cases had been compiled for several decades began to produce collective statistical studies.

Lists of possible etiologies created a opportunity to count the number of cases that fell into each category and to generalize about underlying causes. J. J. Putnam, one of the neurologists commenting on Gray's leptomeningitis case in 1893, had two years earlier published, in the same journal, a study of a group of cases of disseminated sclerosis among the feeble elderly, mostly women (J. J. Putnam 1891). The German neurologist Richard von Krafft-Ebing, later to be well-known for studies in the psychiatry of the sex drive, assembled a comprehensive theoretical account of the origins of *multiple Sklerose* (1895). Thus, papers in the European and American journals noted the association (causal or not) of disseminated sclerosis with infectious diseases (especially syphilis), trauma, hysteria, alcoholism and pregnancy. In the absence of clear evidence that heredity played a part in the transmission of a significant number of cases, physicians did not group multiple sclerosis with imbecility and other forms of social degeneration. There were broad studies of the modes of onset (Mackintosh 1903, eighty cases) or of early manifestations (Palmer 1904, fifty cases) of the disease as physicians attempted to marshal the available data to provide themselves with predictive resources.

One of the origins of public health lay in combining geography and statistics with an understanding of contagion: John Snow's maps of cholera distribution and his successful advice for reducing its incidence (remove the pump handle) became legendary. The first application of this vision of infectious disease to a chronic disease, disseminated sclerosis, is probably in the studies of an energetic Edinburgh practitioner, Byrom Bramwell. Between 1903 and 1905 Bramwell published a series of papers in Edinburgh medical journals — mostly in *Clinical Studies*, which he edited — on the symptomatology, etiology and distribution of cases of the disease. His clinical work is routine for the time, but his observations on the geographical significance of cases were a summary of his own practice and those of many other physicians and case workers in Europe and America. While pursuing precipitating causes, Bramwell arrived at a new conclusion that removed the collective case study of disseminated sclerosis from a strict dependence on categories of causes.

An important influence on Bramwell's thinking was the sheer number of cases he was able to review.

> In my experience, disseminated sclerosis is, comparatively speaking, a common disease in this country [Great Britain]. It certainly seems to be very much more common here than it is in America. I have lately gone through all my hospital and private case-books with the object of determining the actual and relative frequency of the disease. After excluding re-entries and re-admissions I find that I have notes, more or less complete, of 6406 cases of nervous disease (organic and functional), and that in these 6406 cases there were 110 cases of disseminated sclerosis; consequently 1 in every 58 nervous cases was a case of disseminated sclerosis. ... The result of my observations is to show that in this country (Scotland and the North of England) at least 1 out of every 52 cases of nervous disease met with in hospital practice, and at least 1 in every 64 cases of nervous disease met with in private practice, is a case of disseminated sclerosis. Now contrast these figures with the American statistics ... it will be seen that in 8000 private patients observed by Drs. Dana, [Graeme] Hammond, and Sachs, there were 38 cases of disseminated sclerosis — in other words, 1 in every 210 cases of nervous disease in private practice was a case of disseminated sclerosis; while in 32,215 hospital cases observed by Drs. Dana, Hammond, Allen, Starr (Dr. Goodhart), Onuf, Fisher, Collins, and Fraenkel, there were 141 cases of disseminated sclerosis — in other words, 1 in every 221 cases of nervous disease in private practice was a case of disseminated sclerosis. ... My statistics, therefore, seem to show that, taking both private and hospital patients together, disseminated sclerosis is, relative to other forms of nervous disease, *at least three and a half times more frequent in this country than in America....*
>
> The difference is very remarkable. I cannot explain it.

Bramwell offered the first statistically supported generalization about the distribution of disseminated sclerosis. He took care to check the distorting influence of double-counting of patients and the differences caused by varying diagnostic standards from one physician to another or from one time to another ("I admit that I now diagnose some cases as disseminated sclerosis which I would not have diagnosed as disseminated sclerosis ten years ago"). His conclusion of differential distribution between his practice in Scotland and that of the New York doctors is significant for the degree of professional cooperation it required. He has to be confident that what he is calling disseminated sclerosis is what his transatlantic colleagues are calling disseminated sclerosis. His work is one more manifestation of the spread of diagnostic standards that apply to this particular condition. From among thousands of people who have reached neurologists with all manner of complaints, an internationally comparable group of disseminated sclerosis patients can be singled out.

Bramwell does not try to explain his distribution contrast but just adds it to the list of characteristics of the disease. He summarizes the etiology of the disease, using his numbers to support existing observations that the disease is more common among women than among men and that it usually begins in early adult life. He also supports the general conclusion that the disease is not hereditary. He found that single people developed disseminated sclerosis more frequently than those married. Although occupation did not seem to have an influence, the great majority of cases were "comfortably or fairly well circumstanced as regards their home surroundings; only a small proportion were in very poor circumstances." Syphilis and gonorrhea did not seem to play a role in bringing about the disease, and the list of causes either elicited or spontaneously given by patients was quite varied. Febrile and infectious disease, mental worry, chills and injuries came after the largest category, "no apparent or alleged cause."

Evaluating the theory that the lesions are caused by a poison carried through the blood, Bramwell wonders why the grey matter, more richly supplied with blood, is not more affected than the white matter. He favors another theory: that the disease is due to some developmental or congenital defect that predisposes the nervous or neuroglial tissue to irritation. It would follow from this that the disease might often be present in some latent form from childhood and become symptomatic with one of the precipitating causes (infection, trauma) often cited. Bramwell didn't refer to Neff and Klingman's article, but he may have agreed with their conclusion that their case's disease came about through the action of infectious agents on a susceptible system. Their idea of hereditary taint might not be so acceptable to him. The components of a theory of causation, which had been present as early as Cruveilhier and Ollivier d'Angers, were now re-formed amid more concentrated case experience.

Bramwell's geography of disseminated sclerosis was the most visible example of a beginning trend to situate concentrations of cases, a trend made possible by the standardization of the diagnostic instrument. In 1905 R. M. Van Wart published a brief note on the frequency of disseminated sclerosis in the U.S. state of Louisiana. Simply the thought that disseminated sclerosis might have a distinct frequency in one place different from that in another place contributed to the consolidation of the disease concept. Comparison of frequencies could give insight into the nature of the disease.

Bramwell's claim of different frequencies required that anyone accepting the claim believe that he and the American neurologists were finding the same disease. As more cases were reported in and from remote places, a tension inherent in the disseminated sclerosis pathology began to show itself. Charcot had asserted *sclérose en plaques* by showing it was the same as Duchenne's *"parésie choreiforme"* and different from Parkinson's paralysis agitans. Others after him affirmed, criticized or ignored his school's formulation by proposing new or old disease entities behind a case of disseminated sclerosis. The quest for etiologies was an outgrowth of the differential manner in which disseminated sclerosis was defined in the first place. The strong characterization of the disease encouraged communication among physicians who might otherwise have remained isolated with their few cases. Saying that disseminated sclerosis was something else proceeded into saying that something otherwise undefined was *like* disseminated sclerosis. This communicated succinctly the nature of the newly described condition and refined diagnostics. The disease in its Charcotian form was becoming a shared grammatical principle in the developing international language of neurology.

The Salpêtrière-trained Algerian practitioner Georges Scherb, in a later number of that school's ongoing photographic record, *Nouvelle Iconographie de la Salpêtrière*, marked the break in the diagnostics even of those trying to adhere to the old clinical pathology. Scherb (1905a) was uncertain whether his patient was showing the symptoms of *sclérose en plaques* or of what he called *"le syndrome cérébelleux de Babinski."* The familiar tremor and nystagmus, and some additional motor disturbances, might be due to a cerebellum pathology that Babinski had described and not to the distribution of lesions in the cerebellum, which was also being described as a special form of disseminated sclerosis. Scherb asked of another case (1905b) if it was *sclérose en plaques* or *"maladie de Charcot."* Julius Althaus had proposed calling disseminated sclerosis "Charcot's disease" (shorter name) in 1878 (Althaus 1878:330–35), but that designation did not catch on even among Althaus's colleagues in the United States. This later "Charcot's disease" was the subject of several other papers (DeBuck and Demeer 1896; Gallego Moyano 1904), based on Charcot's differentiating from *sclérose en plaques* an atrophy of arm and leg muscles with marked limitation of peripheral nerve sensation (1892: vol. 1, 243–44). Charcot and his associate Pierre Marie published a joint paper (1886), and Marie (1904) and the English neurologist Howard Tooth (1906) each added their observations for Charcot-Marie-Tooth disease to be recognized as a distinct clinical entity, rare but most often occurring in children and probably hereditary. Charcot himself has no single disease named after him; his description of *sclérose en plaques* was not the first or unique.

There had been discussion of disseminated scler*oses* during the years after Charcot's definition (Wood 1878). By the turn of the century, some physicians were diagnosing "combined" multiple sclerosis of both brain and spinal column with dementia, ataxia and other usually unassociated symptoms (Gonzalez 1902; Hunt 1903). New axes of differentiation brought other known pathologies into a comparative relationship with disseminated sclerosis. The emphasis on differential diagnosis reduced the confusion caused by excessive confidence in symptoms.

German and Russian diagnosticians recognized a "*Westphal'sche Pseudosklerose*," after Carl Westphal's studies of children's multiple sclerosis–like brain disease (1888), also known to occur in acute form in adults (Kaplan 1903). Albrecht Strümpell, who had studied the pathological anatomy of the brains of syphilitics and alcoholics, in the late 1890s (1898; 1900) consolidated his findings in a series of articles on "*Pseudosklerose*." Here the living patient has multiple sclerosis symptoms but shows no island lesions at autopsy. Like Landon Gray's leptomeningitis case mimicking disseminated sclerosis, Strümpell's cases were symptomatically multiple sclerosis but did not have multiple sclerosis lesions.

Multiple sclerosis was commonly differentiated from and associated with syphilis, as it became clear that they shared symptoms and syndromes such as ataxias and tabes dorsalis, which in turn might be taken for either of them (e.g., Meirowitz 1900; Sinkler 1902). The phrase "differential diagnosis" in various languages when applied to central nervous system scleroses was virtually a euphemism for providing systematic distinctions between scleroses and syphilis sequels. Children with symptoms of MS might actually have had congenital syphilis or a pseudosclerosis. They tended to show symptoms without pathology more frequently than adults and gave the clearest examples of pseudosclerosis.

In 1879 Strümpell had found that the brain of a lifetime alcoholic was hardened as a mass, a diffuse rather than an islet sclerosis. Other brain pathologies of patients exhibiting multiple sclerosis symptoms showed this general or broadly localized hardening rather than distinct plaques. The term "pseudosclerosis" therefore meant "pseudomultiplesclerosis" and came into usage to describe the diagnostic condition in which the pathology does not correspond to the symptoms. Diffuse sclerosis had been an ill-defined category at the middle of the nineteenth century, when Frerichs mixed several cases with disseminated sclerosis. Those who had the chance to make clinical pathology studies assumed almost a continuum from many separate patches to general hardening. This was taken to explain the great variability of symptoms within the disseminated sclerosis realm and the resemblance of symptoms to those of so many other diseases.

Confusion continued through the work of Hammond, who in attempting to study diffuse and disseminated sclerosis epitomized them symptomatically and made only limited reference to tissues. Westphal, Strümpell and their colleagues (often rivals), focusing microscopically on the cerebral matter itself, distinguished a diffuse sclerosis from a disseminated one. Westphal used the phrase "multiple sclerosis" (same in German) for both kinds; Strümpell used the word "pseudosclerosis" for the deviant cases. No one was sure how much difference there really was between diffuse and multiple localized sclerosis. If they all caused the same range of symptoms, then there must be an underlying similarity on the cellular level beneath the different degrees of hardness.

Oswald Marburg (1905) introduced a phrase to epitomize the pathology of the "so-called acute multiple sclerosis" cases he examined: encephalitis periaxalis scleroticans. "Encephalitis" identified the disease as an inflammation of the brain interior, "periaxalis" specified the neural axons as the site of the inflammation and "scleroticans" delineated the tissue transformation that resulted. Despite its ponderous sound, this label is a minimal designation of multiple sclerosis pathology. It treats that pathology as the concomitant and possibly the result of infection, and leaving aside vascular sites, the term places the nerves and particularly the axons at the center of the disease action. Whatever may be going on symptomatically, this encephalitis has its distinct pathological anatomy. With Marburg's archaic-sounding medical terminology, multiple sclerosis entered the twentieth century.

A precise scientific term suggests a structure with other definable components. Where there was encephalitis periaxalis scleroticans there could be other kinds of encephalitis: encephalitis perimyelitis scleroticans and so on. Paul Schilder (1912) reported the case of a 14-year-old girl who exhibited multiple sclerosis symptoms rapidly culminating in dementia and death; when, in postmortem, he found extensive demyelination over both cerebral hemispheres, he recalled the opportunity created by Marburg's words and named the disease "encephalitis periaxalis diffusa." Schilder's paper refers to the "so-called diffuse scleroses," reflecting the title of Marburg's earlier study and preparing for his own more specific definition.

As C. M. Poser and L. Van Bogaert later recognized (1956), Schilder's diffuse sclerosis, also called Schilder's disease, is the end result of a long evolution that required making distinctions between different kinds of brain scleroses. The brain was a province that Charcot, and therefore many of his students, hesitated to examine. The German tradition of brain pathology led to independent conclusions dissenting from and modifying the Salpêtrière model. In the fine examination of children's brain tissue, Strümpell, Marburg and Schilder sectioned off a pathology that had long been subsumed beneath the rubric of multiple sclerosis (acute multiple sclerosis, pseudosclerosis). Those mysterious adult symptomatic cases that did not show plaques at autopsy might have been due to Schilder's disease, and certainly sudden-onset childhood multiple sclerosis might be understood differently.

Egon Stenager (1992) questioned Schilder's priority of description. The result was a revelation, as has already happened a few times in multiple sclerosis history and can happen a few more. Stenager found that Ludwig Stohr, who died the year Schilder was born (1886), had already described Schilder's disease, though obviously not within the same set of parameters that gave Schilder recognition. There is even cause to wonder whether there really is a disease, Schilder's or not (Cotrufo et al. 1969).

There were concurrent activities of brain assay within Germany. When Friedrich Pelizaeus set down the details of what he called a "unique form of spastic crippling with cerebral manifestations" occurring mainly in children (1885), he immediately compared it with multiple sclerosis, while noting that it had a "hereditary basis." The brain tissue did not show the plaques of multiple sclerosis but extensive hardening over the cerebral hemispheres. Like many other anatomists, Pelizaeus called this "multiple sclerosis" because he believed that there were plaques present but that they were too small even for the microscope to detect. Ludwig Merzbacher (1904), apparently unaware of Pelizaeus's clinical studies, wrote of a familial disease of the central nervous system with symptoms of multiple sclerosis but a diffuse hardening of the tissue and no visible lesions. This diffuse familial sclerosis, or Pelizaeus-Merzbacher disease, provided the decidedly hereditary end to a line that included multiple sclerosis in the less definitely hereditary sector. Taken together, these pathologies outline a chart with separate cells for diffuse vs. multiple (disseminated) sclerosis and hereditary vs. nonhereditary sclerosis. Pelizaeus-Merzbacher filled the hereditary diffuse sclerosis cell, and Schilder's disease filled the nonhereditary diffuse sclerosis cell, but the hereditary multiple sclerosis cell remained unoccupied. This forming chart helped motivate the search for that entity, as if it were an unknown planet exerting a detectable gravity on visible bodies.

Many natural objects (that is, not in themselves created by human beings)—stars and planets, chemical elements, subatomic particles, animals and plant species—have been classified according to plans that predict the presence of as yet undiscovered components. Their discovery then tends to support at least the heuristic value of the classifying scheme already used. Within the subsystem that developed to classify multiple sclerosis, the categories most conspicuously unoccupied by named diseases with cases and cellular pathology are those in the area of heredity and infectious causation. The force of the search is in part impelled by the need to satisfy those categories. Despite the repeated assertions by clinicians that they see very limited hereditary transmission and no consistent infection at the root of MS, there is a constant search to discover heredity and infection in MS.

In a paper delivered before the Southwest German Psychiatric meeting in 1906, later published in 1907 (Bick, Amaducci and Pepeu 1987), Alois Alzheimer presented a single but novel case: a 51-year-old woman who had suffered severe memory loss and disturbances of speech and understanding. With the thoroughness that he had shown in his earlier examinations of brain arteriosclerosis, Alzheimer followed the case through to autopsy and found the woman's brain severely atrophied. Examining the specially stained tissue under the microscope, he saw that the neurofibrils within normal-looking cells had become thickened and in some cells had even replaced the nucleus and cytoplasm. In addition to this pathology in various stages, Alzheimer found "miliary foci ... which represented the sites of deposition of a peculiar substance in the cerebral cortex."

These "miliary plaques" had already been seen in the brains of senile patients and may have been identical with the miliary sclerosis sometimes grouped with incompletely symptomatic disseminated sclerosis. Alzheimer was working in the same milieu as and using pathological tools similar to those of Marburg and Schilder, but unlike them, he did not situate his discovery in relation to the parameters of brain sclerosis (diffuse/multiple) and he did not refer to multiple sclerosis in his conclusions, even as a type or comparison. Alzheimer's neurofibrils and plaques became a strong explanatory tool for a range of senile and pre-senile dementias. The same controversies arose with these miliary cerebral plaques as arose with multiple sclerosis and with the dystrophies: were they the result of proliferation of transformed (glial) cells already there or the result of an introduction of a foreign substance, perhaps an exogenous toxin? Fortunately Alzheimer defied the differential brain sclerosis diagnosis of mental disease and looked carefully at the cells. But multiple sclerosis and its array of counterparts have continued to be clinical and pathological benchmarks: many diseases are defined in reference to multiple sclerosis symptoms and multiple sclerosis pathology. Alfons Jacob (1921) referred to his cases of a "noteworthy" senile dementia as "resembling multiple sclerosis" (*"nahstehende multiple Sklerose"*). He also called it a "spastic pseudosclerosis." The vocabulary of German brain scleroses had to be invoked to introduce a new disorder, with a spongiform pathology that is not a sclerosis at all.

"Multiple sclerosis" came to designate a set of features, symptoms and pathology that could be invoked to assimilate into medical categories something new, whether Creutzfeld-Jakob disease in the 1920s or Lyme disease and chronic fatigue syndrome during the 1980s. Dissemination of the MS concept has continued in this way, as it is used to differentiate (and invent) new diseases.

8

The Realization
of Pathology

A distinctive pathology gave MS its name and the power to define other diseases. As symptomatology became more refined, the symptoms — optic neuritis, speech disturbances — were disease states apart from MS. Pathology remained the one reliable indication. The only way to understand the distinctiveness and thus the development and causes of MS was to know the pathology in all of its details, to see that it was cerebral plaques making the afflicted stumble, blink and slur their speech. The medical history of MS was driven by analysis and imaging of the lesions and by the wish to watch them in the living patient.

The 1906 Nobel prize in physiology and medicine was shared by Santiago Ramón y Cajal and Camillo Golgi. Golgi, the older of the two, had developed a stain that coated the finest nerve fibers and set them visibly apart from other tissue as a lovely silver mesh in the higher magnifications of dark field microscope. Golgi's stain showed him the connections of the brain as a unified whole. Ramón y Cajal used a modification of Golgi's stain to discover the opposite: that the nerves of the brain were physically discontinuous links broken at synapses. Golgi roundly denounced Ramón y Cajal in his Nobel lecture, but Ramón y Cajal's new vision of the cerebral and spinal white matter took its place alongside Golgi's. They both showed the brain as an interconnected mass, though they interpreted the nature of the connections differently.

These preparations were of "normal" brains: it was crucial that the specimens not be diseased. It was a while before the new connective staining methods were systematically applied to the brains of people with neurological disorders. Stains were still being applied to show the location of the damage. The details of pathology were ever better revealed by the continuing development of stains able to pick out specific features.

In 1885 Karl Nissl had announced his method of staining ganglion cells in both normal and diseased tissue. Alois Alzheimer developed further staining methods; like Nissl, he included the overlooked gray matter of the brain in his meticulous studies. In his *Diseases of the Central Nervous System* (1908), Archibald Church still showed MS lesions in drawings of spinal and cerebral sections stained with Weigert's glial stain to reveal the areas of damage. Church described the "round or angular circumscribed spots irregularly disseminated like defects in the nervous substance ... as if they had been pierced with a stiletto." The stain demonstrated that MS is primarily a disease of the nerve support cells called glia and not of the nerve axons or of the blood vessels. This was one opinion in the continuing controversy between those who saw MS as a disease beginning in the blood vessels and those who saw it as a disease beginning in the nerves themselves. Using other stains led to other opinions but always with the same imagery.

In July 1910 Dr. Alexander Bruce, an Edinburgh pathologist, and Dr. J. W. Dawson, a neurological histologist in the Royal College of Physicians laboratory, also in Edinburgh, published a brief communication in the *Proceedings of the Pathological Society of Great Britain and Ireland*. On the basis of a study of MS ("disseminated sclerosis") using Golgi and Ramón y Cajal stains, the investigators suggested that MS is a "toxi-infective disease." The plaques are distributed in relation to the veins and the walls of the ventricles: the toxic substance travels the circulatory system and enters the nerve tissue through the lymphatic channels around the veins and induces plaque formation in those places. This communication favored the vascular theory of MS. Bruce and Dawson had traced the anatomical components of characteristic plaque distribution.

Bruce died shortly before the completion of the report, and Dawson continued the work along the lines they had projected. Six years later he published his massive monograph *The Histology of Multiple Sclerosis* (Dawson 1916). The monograph is an MS compendium on the scale of other late Victorian-Edwardian masterworks: Fraser's *Golden Bough* for beliefs and customs or Pitt-Rivers's museum for material culture. It was not the first work in which photomicrographs were printed to show the stained details of MS lesions, but it certainly was the most extensive ever. There are several hundred photographs among the 456 illustrations, which also include many color drawings of formations that do not show well in printed photos. Improvements in microscope lighting had augmented other design advances to enable Dawson to show visually the results of using the new stains and sectioning methods. "As far as histological methods are concerned it is impossible to expect any further results by their employment," declared one reviewer (*Lancet* 1916: vol. 1, 1090).

Dawson carried forward and vindicated the work he and Bruce had begun eight years earlier. He systematically compared his findings with those of earlier writers, in the process accumulating one of the largest bibliographies of early MS studies. He did not claim to have uncovered the cause or the exact nature of the disease. He did present in considerable detail a six-step pathological process beginning with a simultaneous degeneration of the myelin and reaction of the glia, leading to glial proliferation and fat-granule cell formation. The fat-granule cells are exuded into the nerve tissue, where they interfere with the activities of the nerves. MS is a "subacute encephalo-myelitis" that terminates in areas of permanent sclerosis. What differentiates it from other central nervous system afflictions is the remitting-relapsing symptom pattern. Dawson attributed this to the tendency of the fat-granule cells to clear up even as the nerve tissue is hardening. The axon-cylinders, which carry the nerve impulses, are not themselves affected by the process. The pattern of interference with nerve transmissions would therefore be irregular and sporadic, though most likely slowly progressive.

Dawson continued to support his and Bruce's original argument that a circulating toxin was at the base of MS. It was more likely to be a toxic agent than microbial, transmitted by the blood vessels rather than the lymph system. The anatomical pattern of MS supported a toxin of selective action, which Dawson thought might accumulate slowly and or might be eliminated less efficiently. In all of these suggestions, Dawson tabulated earlier postulates about the cause of MS with microanatomical evidence and set out theories that would be tested over the course of the century.

The strictly physical nature of his evidence made him confident that he had given "approximately final answers ... to the questions relating to the process underlying disseminated sclerosis, to its origin, to the relation of several secondary etiological factors, and to certain aspects of the mode of action of the final causal agent." He emphasized: "We are still in the dark concerning the nature of this final cause, which determines, anatomically, a process so well defined and one without any close analogy. ... All that is most important still remains for future investigations along bacteriological, serological, and experimental lines."

Dawson's work was the culmination of the previous century's discoveries and biases. He presented a static anatomy animated in stages of disease progression through the study of different tissue samples in relation to each other. That so many MS tissue samples were available to Dawson and others at this time results from the growing ability to detect the disease and follow patients through to autopsy.

E. W. Taylor (1922:564) described Dawson's correlation between symptoms and anatomy as "dogmatic." Weakness in the legs developing into paralysis, Dawson wrote, "is obviously the clinical manifestation of the dense areas of sclerosis which were found throughout the spinal cord." And so on he continued through a long list of correlations between symptoms and plaque locations. Dawson's anatomical skills enabled him to determine the age of a lesion, which could then be related to the nature and seriousness of a symptom observed before the patient's death: nystagmus, eye flickering early in the disease, "undoubtedly" was the result of patches around the brain ventricles, patches that were shown to be old at autopsy.

Dawson's anatomical demonstrations were quite influential. Anatomical studies like that of Theophil Klingman (1919) are indebted to Dawson's account of the pathological process. Klingman even includes an intricate drawing that summarizes several of the illustrations of process in Dawson's book. Klingman does not refer to Dawson, perhaps because the reference would have been commonly understood among specialists. His account of the components of the process is different from Dawson's, and several other differences in detail obscure the overall similarity. Over the years Dawson's process became a framework for guiding the view of stained lesion anatomy at the middle level of magnification.

Yet as Taylor's objections indicate, Dawson's account of the relationship between symptoms and anatomy was not so readily accepted, which in turn tended to cast doubt on the usefulness of his anatomy. Dawson's anatomical precision and the demonstrable imprecision of symptom correlates (the spasms rarely occurred as predicted from the anatomy) subverted the exact relation between lesion location and symptom type, a relation that had been current since Charcot.

The neuropathologist Barends Brouwer (1920) offered an alternative theory that looked to the evolution of the central nervous system. Brouwer wondered why some MS patients lose the ability to speak while not suffering any loss of cranial nerve function. Why does the eye always jerk from side to side in nystagmus and not up and down? In optic neuritis, why does only one part of the optical disk pale while the entire optic nerve is affected? Brouwer proposed that the older parts of the central nervous system, the cranial nerves for instance, are more likely to be able to resist an infectious agent (the cause of MS) than are the newer parts, such as the speech function. The horizontal motion of the eyes is newer than the vertical, and so on. The "age" of nerve components in humans is determined by comparative anatomy: animals have cranial nerves, but they don't have speech centers in the brain, which are a human specialization.

There are objections to this evolutionary account of MS, on several grounds; for example, there is no guarantee that MS is caused by an infectious agent. Brouwer's account does mark a trend away from the symptomatics that Dawson laid the groundwork for in his anatomy. Dawson believed that tracing the anatomy of MS lesions ever more finely would provide a finer map of the outward symptoms. But there was reason to doubt that. Even if you could look into the brain and spine at precise points, you could not see the nerve failures that caused vertigo, eye problems and urinary incontinence in the patient. It was not possible to establish simple correspondence between a site in the normal brain and an action of the body; it was equally difficult to demonstrate correspondences between diseased tissue and particular symptoms.

Dawson was more an heir of Charcot than the anatomists who followed him were his heirs. The middle magnification, stained anatomy became the ground for the search for microbial agents and for experimentation. Dawson's work was the "last word" in MS histology. Those who followed accumulated more detail and balanced the significance of one feature against another. By 1933 George Hassin, in his *Histopathology of the Peripheral and Central Nervous System*, made only passing mention of Dawson, and in his note on "The Rise of Neuropathology" in the first volume of the *Journal of Neuropathology and Experimental Neurology* Hassin (1942) mentioned Charcot, Nissl, Alzheimer, Golgi and Ramón y Cajal but not Dawson. Dawson had not invented anything but had merely applied the methods of others, with dedication.

Experimentation with animals was a way to try to see into the living brain to detect the changes that accompany the manifestations of paralysis and other symptoms. But even with animals, it was not possible to view the tissue changes as they occurred; an animal could live only so long with its brain exposed. As Brouwer's speculations reminded experimenters, there are significant differences between the structures of human brains and those of dog brains. The experiments could be valid only to observe generalized nerve tissue effects. But there were other reasons to pursue animal experiments.

The possibility of a technological innovation that would allow a peek into the living brain emerged with the development of medical X-ray photography early in the twentieth century. Pathologists had fantasized a photography that could penetrate the skull without harming the subject. X-ray photographs could show the breaks in bones and the spots of tuberculosis on the lungs. With the proper use of stains, they could even show details of the vascular system in living beings. As an understanding of how to take and how to read X-rays became in itself a medical specialty, some features of brain pathology could be discerned in living people. For a time it was joked that a patient would have to be dead or in seizures before an X-ray showed the brain condition. X-rays were of limited usefulness to surgeons because they presented a flat image whereas the brain is a three-dimensional solid in which each layer is of medical significance. The solid mass of the tumor (or the bullet) would appear only in relation to the walls of the skull and to some shadowy contiguous features that had to be expertly interpreted. There was little chance of making out the exact positioning of the fine lesions of MS. The vision achieved in a postmortem was not available through X-rays of a living brain. The X-ray was not the living image of MS pathology.

The ideal image of the MS brain was what the pathologist saw in an autopsy section. These sectional images were the photographic version of the preserved specimen collections that most medical museums have maintained to this day. Photographs of the sectionally sliced brain (tomographs) appeared along with the photomicrographs in Dawson's compendium and in many others since then. With the perfection of color photography and color offset printing, medical atlases could offer a photographic version of Carswell's or Cruveilhier's colored tomographic lithographs. There have even been color atlases specifically depicting MS tissues.

For X-rays to live up to their potential for making photographs of brain sections, it was necessary to have the massive data-processing capabilities of the computer. By taking X-ray photographs of the brain of a stationary patient from many different positions and computer generating a three dimensional model of the brain, it was possible to produce tomographs, flat images of sections cut in almost any plane. Considerable testing was still required to establish how to resolve MS plaques tomographically in the brains of living patients (Gyldensted 1976). Computer tomography finally realized a living image of MS pathology, at least of the disposition of plaques. This also opened the opportunity to trace changes in plaque concentration and in the dimensions of the brain ventricles.

Within a few years after the maturing of computer-assisted tomographic scanning a completely different method of imaging — magnetic resonance imaging (MRI) — became available. This employs shifts in the intensity of a magnetic field induced around the patient's body to alter the nuclear magnetic resonance of water molecules. Data processing of fluctuations in the field yields a black and white map of tissue densities in any selected part of the body. Adaptation and techniques of interpretation made magnetic resonance images another way of visualizing MS in the brain and spine (Young et al. 1981). MRI also provided tomographic images of the brain and spine. As they became available in color, though not the actual colors of the tissues, they approached the standard that the early anatomical lithographers had created for autopsy findings 150 years earlier. The great difference was that these electromagnetic images could be used to aid in the diagnosis of living people and to follow the changes in their tissues.

No matter how sophisticated the imaging became, it was still confined to the level of the naked eye. Dawson's low-magnification pathology was not available for living tissue. Ever finer optical microscopes and eventually the electron microscope looked more deeply into the specimen tissue. Coupled with improving biochemistry, theories of how molecules behave in the living brain were developed out of analysis and experimentation. But this was a matter of applying more general ideas to MS and other diseases. Anatomy and pathology have not yet entirely dissolved into chemistry. The organ level at which MS was first detected remains the field in which MS is caused and treated.

As technology improved the capacity to gather information by penetrating the living nerves down to ever finer levels of magnification, the highest level of MS became conscious.

9

The Great War

W. N. P. Barbellion (1984) wrote:

A Jolt

Yesterday the wind was taken out of my sails. Racing along with the spinnaker and jib, feeling pretty fit and quite excited over some interesting ectoparasites just collected on some Tinamous, I suddenly shot into a menacing dead calm: that stifling atmosphere which precedes a Typhoon. That is to say, my eye caught the title of an enormous quarto memoir in the *Trans. Roy. Soc.*, Edinburgh: The Histology of _____
_____.

I was browsing in the library at the time when this hit me like a carelessly handled gaff straight in the face. I almost ran away to my room.

Barbellion does not say that he looked at Dawson's *Histology of Multiple Sclerosis*. Like many other aspects of his *Journal of a Disappointed Man* [1919 (1984)], the incident is ambiguous. As a naturalist, he surely would have been interested in the fine tissue structure of his own disease as shown in the photomicrographs accompanying Dawson's text. Yet his terror of peering into his own skull as he had looked into the innards of so many animals ("dissecting my way up and down the animal kingdom") is an understandable terror for a naturalist diagnosed with disseminated sclerosis.

As with many of the personal names in his journal and diary, Barbellion never wrote the words "disseminated sclerosis," and he refers or avers to it infrequently even as he is dying of its symptoms. Even his own name is a pseudonym, taken from the name of a confectioner's shop ("suitably grand") and prefixed with the names of three historical fiends ([Kaiser] Wilhelm, Nero and Pilate). His is the first personal account of the effects of the disease. It marks the first time that someone aware he had disseminated sclerosis published an

account of his life before and during the disease. Yet that was not the purpose
of the book.

Barbellion included entries in his journal from when he was 13 (January 3, 1903) up to the moment of his death, fictionally placed on December 31, 1917, at the end of the *Journal*, but actually occurring on October 22, 1919, a few months short of his 31st birthday. A *Last Diary* is set between March 21, 1918, and June 3, 1919. That he composed *A Last Diary* after his supposed death date (it was published posthumously in 1920 with a short biography by Barbellion's brother A. J. Cummings) indicates his eagerness to make public his impressions and views even at the cost of dissolving the romantic fiction of his death at the end of the 1917. But his motive was not only to achieve a measure of literary fame for a life disappointed of other glories; he also wanted his wife and young daughter to have some revenue.

On December 6, 1914, a week after Barbellion proposed to his future wife (a shadowy figure except for his emotions toward her), he lists the projects he has in mind:

(1) To make her happy and make myself worthy.
(2) To get married.
(3) To prepare and publish a volume of this Journal.
(4) To write two essays for *Cornhill* which shall surely induce the editor to publish and not write me merely long and complimentary letters as heretofore.

The next day he is exclaiming over the number of projects he has in view and the small amount of time he has, over how he is haunted by the fear that he may never complete them "thro' physical or temperamental disabilities." His love and marriage plans, his drive to publish a version of his journal and his physical disability are mingled from this first mention of publishing the journal.

There are other drives present around this love-fearing disability. On December 9 he tells how a passion for symphonic music has replaced his former cravings to study natural history. He implicitly compares himself to a horse: while in the country, he wore only blinkers and saw only zoology. "Now in London, I've taken the bit into my mouth — and it's a mouth of iron — wanting a run for all my troubles before Death strikes me down. All this evidence of temperamental instability alarms and distresses me on reflection and makes the soul weary."

On December 14 he looks over his rooms and sees a litter of "old concert programmes and the Doctor's prescriptions (in the yellow envelopes of the dispenser) for my various ailments and diseases, and books, books, books." He lists some of the books currently on his table: plays, novels, philosophy and Marie Bashkirtseff's *Journal*. He has read only the first chapter of

Bashkirtseff's book and is afraid to go on. "It would be so humiliating to find I was only her duplicate." At one time Barbellion said his father was Sir Thomas Browne (the skeptical physician) and his mother was Marie Bashkirtseff.

Bashkirtseff, of Russian nobility and a painter exhibited in the Paris Salon, died of consumption at the age of 24 in 1884, and her posthumously published *Journal* was a literary sensation in French and English translation. It is the extremely self-absorbed chronicle of her sufferings and her efforts to live life to the fullest amid them, as if the suffering intensified the living. She is Saint Lidwina giving her own story rather than relying on manipulative chroniclers. The figure of Bashkirtseff appealed to Barbellion as a model for turning his own suffering into literature and for a pathetic success too late to enjoy. "It would be difficult in the world's history to discover any two persons with temperaments so alike," he wrote (October 14, 1914) on discovering Matilde Blind's English translation of Bashkirtseff's published journal.

The earlier sections of the *Journal* detail the glorious naturalist wanderings in the countryside, the ill health and visions of death, the egoism and egotism ("As an Egotist [referring to the novel by George Meredith] I hate death because I should cease to be," July 14, 1912). As H. G. Wells notes in his preface, the *Journal* develops from the "fussy egotism" of the earlier half. During this era, egotism was an intellectual movement asserting the primacy of individual tastes and awareness over convention and standardized beliefs.

A paragraph later Barbellion is referring to people who gained consolation from the notoriety of their own decease. "Heine, after a life of sorrow, died with a sparkling witticism on his lips." He envisions his own "immediate decease — an unobtrusive passing away of a rancorous, disappointed, morbid, and self-assertive entomologist in a West Kensington Boarding House — what a mean little tragedy!" Certainly not a death up to the standards of Heine.

The mean, decidedly unromantic death that Barbellion envisioned for himself (and which he never compared with the deaths of the insects he studied — it is a way to Kafka) is in contrast to the deaths of the heroic losers that populated late-nineteenth- and early-twentieth-century British culture, from Gordon falling beneath the waves of Muslim fanatics at Khartoum to Robert Scott, whose death, after narrowly missing being the first to reach the South Pole, Barbellion learned of on February 10, 1913 ("News of Scott's great adventure! Scott dead a year ago!!"). Scott was the last of these national martyrs to be popularized before World War I gave the story a different twist. On November 19, 1914, Barbellion even imagines himself as Scott "writing his last words amid Antarctic cold and desperation." The image of the abandoned freezing martyr dying, pen in hand, referred both to his ambitions and to the physical cold he actually felt.

On January 22, 1913, Barbellion remarks that he lives in a bigger, dirtier city than London — ill health. "Ill health, when chronic, is like a permanent ligature around one's life." At the same time he remarks that he has so much energy that if he were well, he'd "blow the roof off."

Barbellion is one of the first to tell the personal story of a chronic illness. Like his model Marie Bashkirtseff, he is a vital being who is being restrained by the disease and not a malingering sufferer. Barbellion does not include himself among the diseased, moping characters of literature or history. His disease is an obstacle to his outpouring of energy and the completion of his life's projects. Comparing Barbellion with Denton Welch, invalided in an accident at age 20 and the author of a journal on his tribulations, Deborah Singmaster (Barbellion 1984: Introduction) calls him "virile" against Welch's "effete."

The virility does not affect the disease so much as the disease seems to undermine the virility. The true nature of the disease is a constant, underlying fear. On July 6, 1912, he relates that his doctor brought in a specialist because of a spot found on Barbellion's lung, but the diagnosis turns out not to be consumption. But on April 26, 1913, in an entry headed "Two Months' Sick Leave," he is in a horrible panic because he believes he is developing "locomotor ataxy." He notes: "One leg, one arm, and my speech are affected, i.e. the right side and my speech center. M — —[his doctor] is serious. I hope the disease, whatever it is, will be sufficiently lingering to enable me to complete my book." "Locomotor ataxy" was one medical phrase for the symptoms of advanced syphilis. The "well-known nerve specialist Dr H — —," during Barbellion's visit to the doctor on April 30, can find no symptoms of a definite disease, but asks him "suspiciously" if he has ever been with women.

A virile self-assertion might have been the ultimate cause of the debilitating disease, but Barbellion does not say how he answered that question and never refers to sexual adventures. This may be due to his wish to appear an innocent in love and to avoid the censorship that might follow full revelations or to avoid the lack of publication that might precede them. When George Mair, a colleague of Barbellion's brother Hal Cummings at the *Manchester Guardian*, placed the typed manuscript with the publisher Collins, the publisher backed out after beginning to set the book because of the fear of the effect on its school-text business. Barbellion admits that he "rewrote, edited and bowdlerized" his actual journal, which evidently included leaving out his answer to the neurologist's question but not leaving out the question itself. He never mentions the possibility of syphilis, but some of his descriptions suggest that it was alive in his mind.

On October 13, 1913, he reports that he visited a Harley Street oculist "about the sight of one eye, which has caused a lot of trouble and worry of late and continuously haunted me with the possibility of blindness." The specialist reassures him that there is no neuritis but that "the adjustment muscles have been thrown out of gear by the nervous troubles last spring." It is not clear that the specialist believed ocular adjustment muscles are so like fine mechanisms that they can lose their calibration. His metaphor told Barbellion that at least the visual symptoms of syphilis were not beginning to assert themselves. Immediately afterward, Barbellion is once again ruminating his proposal of marriage and proclaiming that he has neither health nor wealth to pursue it.

It presents an inaccurate picture of the *Journal* and *Diary* to dwell on the development of Barbellion's illness, ignoring his natural history excursions, his work as a journalist, his attempts to escape his uncultured small town and his displays of character traits out of keeping with the image of the earnest man kept down by illness. His slanderous remarks on Jews stand out, but they may be part of uprushes of aggressiveness sometimes directed against humanity as a whole. "Others I hate and loathe — for no particular reason," he writes in an entry on October 29, 1913. And he instances an acquaintance "concerning whom I know nothing at all. He may be Jew, Gentile, Socinian, Preadamite, Anabaptist, Rosicrucian — I don't know and I don't care, for I hate him. I should like to smash his face in. I don't know why." He then launches on a fantasy of his violent intentions toward this man's face. On the same day he is reporting his friendship with a depraved, boorish man who thinks Barbellion has consumption. The next day Barbellion is celebrating his own flesh after the morning bath: "The cool, pink skin — I could eat it!" It seems that Barbellion provided the multiple sclerosis behavioral model that Douglas Firth was trying to find an earlier version of in d'Esté.

But the suspicion of consumption has been implanted, and Barbellion's persistent cough brings him back to the doctor, who rules against it ("More Irony," December 13, 1913). "I always just escape: I always almost get something, go somewhere. I have dabbled in a number of diseases but never get one downright — but only enough to make me feel horribly unfit and very miserable without the consolation of being able to regard myself as the heroic victim of some incurable disorder. Instead of being [Robert Louis] Stevenson with tuberculosis I've been Jones with dyspepsia." With fears of blindness and what he calls "heart attacks," Barbellion continues scorning humanity, being restored by art, flirting with his love and missing his disease: "Doctor's Consulting Rooms — my life has been spent in them!"

An accident in late August 1915, in which he slightly concussed his spine, brings a return of the 1913 trouble but on the left rather than the right side: "paralysis and horrible vertigo and presentiments of sudden collapse as I walk." Making his way to the doctor on his twenty-sixth birthday, he learns that it is common to bruise the coccyx and he need not be concerned. Though he hobbles down the road to see the damage done by the bombs during a zeppelin raid, he is too feeble to walk into town to buy a wedding ring for his wedding the next day.

In the third part of the *Journal*, entitled "Marriage," he lists, on November 8, the progression of events:

> Concussion of the spine.
> Resulting paralysis of the left leg ten days before marriage.
> Zeppelin raid (heard a cannon go off for the first time).
> Severe cold in the head day before marriage (and therefore wild anxiety).
> Successful marriage with abatement of cold.
> Return to our home.
> Ten days later, down with influenza.
> A second Zeppelin raid.
> Bad heart attack.
> Then flat sub-let and London evacuated.

> ...How I envy all these men who are participating in this War — soldiers, sailors, war correspondents — all who live and throb and are not afraid. I am a timid youth, anaemic, wearing spectacles, and am frightened by a Zep raid! How humiliating! I hate myself for a white-livered craven: I am suffocated for want of more life and courage.

"Heart attack" is Barbellion's own expression for cardiac arrhythmia, racing and slowing beat, and does not mean a cardiac infarction. He fully participates in the vigorous zest of the war's beginning and does not seem to question it. He is disgusted with the limitations imposed by his body and preventing him from joining in this manly enterprise.

His visit to the recruiting office on November 27, 1915, is "a matter of form under pressure from the authorities." He carries a sealed note from his doctor to show to the examining physician, a doctor already familiar with his case. The note turns out to be unnecessary because he is rejected as soon as his heart is stethoscoped. On the train returning to his country home, he opens the certificate out of curiosity.

> "Some 18 months ago," it ran, "Mr. Barbellion shewed the just visible symptoms of——— ———" and altho' this fact was at once communicated to my relatives it was withheld from me and M —— therefore asked the M.O. to respect this confidence and to reject me without stating on what grounds. He went on to refer to my patellar and plantar reflexes, by which time I had enough, tore the paper up and flung it out the window.
>
> I then returned to the Museum intending to find out what ——— ———was in Clifford Allbutt's System of Medicine. I wondered whether it was brain or heart; and the very thought gave me palpitation. I hope it is heart — something short and sharp rather than lingering. But I believe it must be ———of the brain, the opposite process of softening occurring in old age.

There is no indication in the sequel that Barbellion actually did read Risien Russel's section on disseminated sclerosis in Allbutt. Soon afterward, he is wondering if his wife, E. (his distant cousin Eleanor Benger, a talented fashion designer), knows what he has, as his brothers evidently do. He continues to wonder this until, on November 6, he learns that E. has known all along and that his doctor warned her not to marry him. On November 17 he relays the state of E.'s emotions during the months between learning of the disease and his learning of it himself: "This white hot secret in her bosom as a barricade to perfect intimacy ... then Zeppelin raids and a few symptoms began to grow obvious, until what before she had to take on trust from the Doctor came diabolically true before her eyes." The nature of the disease or the state of anyone else's knowledge of it (even his own) is soon absorbed into his greater struggle to hold on to vitality and have prospects of a future.

He footnotes the entry for September 2, 1916, in which he celebrates his more comfortable health despite colds and unpleasant nerve symptoms, describing the zoological projects he has in view. "Considerately enough this great Crab lets go of my big toe when I am sunk low in health, yet pinches devilishly hard as now when I am well." He uses the little pains of the disease to convey the accompanying mental state. The note leads to the next entry, the jolt he receives on seeing Dawson's *Histology* while running at a strong clip, and on September 24 the report of his fear that his mental powers are disintegrating and that his sensibility is becoming so numbed that, oxlike, he is not aware of his own plight.

But there now surrounds him another framework of concern. On September 26 he shows for the first time awareness that there is going to be a baby and voices his worry about being "paralysed with a wife and child and no money — ugh!" As E. herself goes into childbirth, which he scarcely acknowledges, and she finally discloses to him that she Knows, he praises her courage. The suspicion that the Zeppelin raids brought out visible symptoms is one aspect of his general denunciation of the war; and when a draft notice arrives, he has none of his former heroic fantasy.

He returns to blame the concussion of the spine he had in 1915, saying that it "re-awakened activity among the bacteria." The idea that bacteria might be behind it is a notion he could have acquired from his own doctor, since the syphilitic origin of disseminated sclerosis was a current notion in the medical profession at that time. A further hint that he still suspects a syphilitic base to his disease is in the comfort he derives from the death of Baudelaire from advanced neurosyphilis. On December 12 he recounts an incident, toward the end of September, when E. was being attended while giving birth to their child. Barbellion was feeling so miserable that the nurse sent for the doctor, whom he shows a copy of the certificate of his London doctor (he is careful to note that though he tore up the original, he had a copy made to show to the military examiner). The doctor asks him if it is certain about the disease ("you are very young for it") and puts him through "the usual tricks" of the reflex exam. The doctor advises him to leave at once (a birth attendant's advice to an expectant father) and tells him his wife is all right, setting to rest his contagion fears that must have arisen from his bacterial notion.

In addition to the courses of arsenic and strychnine prescribed to give him some relief, he admits to having tried at different times electrotherapy and homeopathic remedies, behind the back of the medical profession. "I could write a book on the Doctors I have known and the blunders they have made about me" (echoes of d'Esté, whose manuscript was not yet discovered). At the same time he shows signs of becoming an amateur expert in his own disease. He summons a local doctor and presents his symptoms, which the doctor diagnoses. During a conversation Barbellion tells him about Dawson's *Histology* and, after the doctor leaves, says he is "very amiable, very polite — an obvious *non possumus.*" "No, we can't" is an echo of the inability of doctors to do anything about the disease, whatever they know.

On January 20, 1917, he describes himself:

> I am over six feet high and thin as a skeleton; every bone in my body, even the neck vertebrae, creak at odd intervals when I move. So that I am not only a skeleton but a badly articulated one to boot. If this is coupled with the fact of creeping paralysis, you have the complete horror. Even as I sit and write millions of bacteria are gnawing away at my precious spinal cord, and if you put your ear to my back the sound of the gnawing I dare say could be heard.

Barbellion's final physical definition of his illness is an active state of bacterial attack that easily shifts into a metaphor of being eaten away. He knows of Dawson and Russell and has had the analysis of his physicians, but he prefers a personal sentience that ascribes his state to the animal world and treats himself as a pathology specimen, a skeleton not properly prepared but exhibited just the same. This first autobiography to incorporate disseminated sclerosis also incorporates its history, with the author conceiving himself as a specimen, an electric body, an anatomical diagram and an invalid. Zeppelin bombings and a spinal concussion, the physical trauma that many believed precipitate disseminated sclerosis, were for him the initiating effects. A new image for the process of the disease is the parasitism he himself had so much studied as an entomologist. This thought is so fixed in his mind that when he sees his infant daughter nursing at her mother's breast, he compares her to a parasite taking blood and to the asp at the breast of Cleopatra. But then he turns the problem back on himself: "The fact that such images arise shows how rotten to the core I am." He is the parasite who might sap away his wife's life with his invalid demands.

Barbellion is exquisitely sensitive to his own ability to make his record. He compares his pen as it moves over the paper of the journal to a delicate needle point "tracing out a graph of temperament so as to show its daily fluctuations: grave and gay, up and down, lamentation and revelry, self-love and self-disgust." This is another personal resolution of the impersonal medical history of the disease up to this point. The pen point of the tremor-graphing devices that Charcot and other students of nervous disorders used to chart the muscular movements of patients has, in Barbellion's shaking hand (or through his dictation), become an instrument to describe the inward state of those fluctuating lines. Whether the evocation of that device is deliberate or not, Barbellion has fleshed out the mechanical. The involuntary and spontaneous changes in tremor are meshed with his changes in mood.

This is an instrumental instance of what recurs fleshed out in different ways throughout the *Journal* and the *Last Diary*: treating objects as mood forms of his disease, whether the object is an illustration of Archaeopteryx in an encyclopedia, a swallow outside his window, his gastrocnemius muscle, the journal itself—which as Barbellion becomes more "static and moribund becomes more active and aggressive"—or his little canary ("I too am an animal and we both must die"). As he becomes more bed-bound and dependent, the rush of images and the changes of mood become faster and ferocious. He refers to his twinges, pangs and spasms that interrupt his relentless analytical brain. He has recourse to laudanum, though not as much as he would like. Left alone in the cottage, he climbs upstairs to find a bottle of laudanum but is so slow that his wife returns before he can recover it. He makes up a story, but he knows that she knows what he was looking for.

Barbellion never ceases to evoke the nature that surrounds him and filled his childhood adventures recorded in the earlier part of the journal. The rushing about and mingling of living things and their susceptibility to both precise and impressionistic description are his sense of the world around him. His *Last Diary*, occupied with the literary fate of the *Journal*, comments on current writers, especially James Joyce, whose *Dubliners* he greatly appreciated and whose *Ulysses* causes him to exclaim: "Damn! It's all my idea, the technique I projected." Both Joyce and Barbellion read Henri Bergson, and they were not the only ones to do so. But Barbellion then proclaims that the naturalists are ahead of the novelists, and he celebrates the exhaustive detail of recording in works by Edmund Selous and Julian Huxley. For Barbellion, stream of consciousness is a stream of minutiae observed and rendered.

On the next day (March 16, 1918) he reports getting rapidly worse. "One misery adds itself to another as I explore the course of this hideous disease." On October 5, 1918, he is stirred by the prospect of a cure (as we all have been at one time or another): a London neurologist has injected a serum into the spine of an ailing woman ("and as her disease is the same as mine they wish me to try it too"). He rejoices in the possibility of being able to walk and write again, have his life prolonged. But we never again hear of the cure. Instead, it is the stream of misery.

On March 17, 1918, he evokes Hector Berlioz and quotes Berlioz's "amazing Memoirs writing to a friend for forgiveness for causing him anxiety."

> But you know how my life fluctuates. One day calm, dreary, rhythmical; the next bored, nerve-torn, snappy and surly as a mangy dog; vicious as a thousand devils, sick of life and ready to end it, were it not for the frenzied happiness that draws ever nearer, for the odd destiny that I feel is mine; for my staunch friends; for music, and lastly for *curiosity*. This *verfluchte* curiosity! I could botanise over my own grave, attentively examine the maggots out of my own brain.

Up to the end, at least to the end of his journal keeping, Barbellion was examining not maggots but ctenophors: "The brightest thing in the world is a ctenophor in a glass jar standing in the sun." A collection of essays and stories, published after his death to earn some money for his wife and child while his name remained known, was entitled *Enjoying Life and Other Literary Remains*.

Barbellion's works were not treated as autobiography by reviewers but as a literary journal, and as such, they were widely praised for their authenticity and vitality. The historian A. F. Pollard did take Barbellion to task in the April 1921 issue of *History*, questioning especially the accuracy of some of his references to the events of World War I, as a veteran would of a noncombatant. The books seem to have created a strong-enough image of the life of a sufferer from disseminated sclerosis for Douglas Firth, commenting on Augustus d'Esté, to make a point of d'Esté's few natural history observations (the barred legs of the Aedes mosquito), as if the nineteenth century d'Esté in retrospect had to live up to a standard later set by Barbellion.

Barbellion's special place as the author of the first published personal account of his own disseminated sclerosis may have been an item of common knowledge among British physicians even though seldom commented on, but it is more likely that a continuing literary interest in Barbellion's life and writings (rather than in his natural history researches) maintained his presence for anyone interested to associate him with the disease. The *Journal* has remained in print in Great Britain until the present day, entering its seventh printing in 1923, being printed in Chatto and Windus's popular Phoenix Library in 1931 and going through several printings as a paperback and as a deluxe literary hardbound since then. It is not mentioned even in detailed histories of twentieth century British literature, though Barbellion is listed in biographical indices and in the *Encyclopædia Britannica*. When W. I. McDonald mentioned Barbellion, together with d'Esté, in his article on multiple sclerosis in the *Cambridge World History of Human Disease* (1993:883), it was the first time an active medical researcher had associated Barbellion's name with the disease in print. The subsequent stories of Barbellion's wife, Eleanor Benger, and of his daughter are still to be traced.

There have been numerous multiple sclerosis autobiographies since Barbellion's death and even more biographies and autobiographies that include mention of multiple sclerosis. Few have achieved Barbellion's intensity of self-knowledge in the midst of the disease, perhaps because despite his declared egotism (or egoism), he craved to be aware of the natural world outside its umbra.

Disseminated sclerosis in Barbellion's *Journal* is a transformation of the narrator of those finely observed natural histories of the British countryside, from Gilbert White's *Natural History of Selborne* to John White's *The Red Deer*. Barbellion is trying to look outward and study living creatures, but he cannot ignore the failure of his own body and he suspects the reasons in the midst of the doctors' veiled speculations. He was primarily a taxonomist and anatomist; the joyous visions of life he saw were not reflected in his classifying technical science. B. F. Cummings's natural history papers do not gaze at animals living among themselves. Like other naturalists of his time Barbellion for the most part ignored natural selection and ecology and concentrated on the tabulation of specimens, ironically similar to what physicians were doing with cases of neurological disease at the same time.

W. H. Hudson was publishing his natural history studies of English settings during the years of Barbellion's youth, and in 1918, at the age of 77, happened to publish his own autobiography, *Long Ago and Far Away*, which recalls his youth exploring the pampas of Argentina where he grew up. Barbellion must have been aware of Hudson but does not mention him at all.

The bank officer Kenneth Grahame, whose only published book is the children's classic *The Wind in the Willows* (1908), originally composed for his young son, seems closer to Barbellion in his evocation of animal life as a long idyll governed by its own distinct etiquette and troubled only by the eccentricities of the animals themselves. Grahame was a Barbellion free of his disease and beset only by the inability of memory to re-create entirely the natural world remembered from his childhood — except, of course, Barbellion dissected his animals and worked in a museum, not a bank.

Despite Pollard's criticism, Barbellion was not isolated from the war going on in Europe. He rose up patriotically at first but then soured on the dreary, wasteful, murderously destructive grind, as did his contemporaries Richard Aldington, Robert Graves, Sigfried Sassoon and e.e. cummings (no relation). Barbellion maintained a traumatic theory of the disease, blaming the pounding of the explosives dropped by Zeppelins for his worst relapse and generally cursing the deprivations and relocations caused by the war.

World War I advanced the medical specialty of war trauma on several fronts. Specialists like Purves-Stewart turned to studies of neurological disease to find an explanation for the reactions they encountered in soldiers. Psychologists and psychiatrists reaped a grim harvest of testimonies of the effects of sustained terror, mass confusion and incessant noise. The field of MS psychiatry became established in the years after the war.

Barbellion's life and death with MS were personal history that went beyond boyhood reminiscences and stories of suffering. MS was no longer described only in medical case histories. With its colorings of infectious disease and invalidism, MS was another war being fought.

10

Epidemics

Barbellion, for all his egotism, was one person with MS among uncounted others. In the years after the war, these people were being counted.

Any historical increase in the rate of multiple sclerosis would be very difficult to prove. Because death statistics are the earliest and most efficiently collected statistics, most of the early epidemiological studies of multiple sclerosis relied on mortality numbers. In the early 1920s the impression that multiple sclerosis cases were clustered geographically gave rise to a number of prevalence studies. (*Prevalence* is the number of active cases of a disease in a population at any one time.)

R. Bing and H. Reese (1926) surveyed four cantons in the northwest of Switzerland and found the prevalence of multiple sclerosis to be measurably higher than in other parts of Europe but also to be highly irregular among the cantons. They had little data for wider comparison, but they did observe that there was an increase in prevalence in the north over the south. Over the next 75 years, three more prevalence studies were conducted in Switzerland, each one taking advantage of the increasing comprehensiveness and efficiency of Swiss clinical medicine to generate ever more supportable numbers for all 25 cantons and confirming many of Bing and Reese's initial conclusions. The advantage of prevalence studies over mortality counts is that disease onset was usually recorded in a clinic, where it was more likely that doctors seeing the living patient would make a correct diagnosis.

Because epidemiology counts cases that already have been diagnosed, it represents a further remove from individual medicine and toward statistical generalities appropriate to a state-organized treatment of disease. This is a movement from a medical conception of multiple sclerosis to a public-health conception. The earliest surveys, in Switzerland and Northern Ireland (Allison 1931), were performed where centralized state authority was uncertain. These surveys depended on local medical practitioners to identify the multiple sclerosis cases. They paralleled other aspects of central authority in requiring the understanding and cooperation of local clinicians to achieve the general purpose.

Case ascertainment and multiple sclerosis epidemiology depended on knowing that each case counted was in fact a multiple sclerosis case. If individual diagnosis of MS was difficult because MS resembles so many other conditions, epidemiology might be equally difficult because names and standards vary. Before the varying rates of multiple sclerosis can be explained, the rates have to measure actual cases.

From Bramwell's early enumerations onward, apparent clusters of multiple sclerosis cases were being declared and even explained without a guarantee that all these cases were authentic. The history of MS epidemiology turns on case ascertainment, just as the history of MS as a disease entity turns on diagnosis. Concentrations of MS cases could be due to factors other than hidden causes of MS. Leonard Kurland points to a study of eight cases of MS in a small New England town; the cases attracted interest because their number was all out of proportion for the population size. Seven of the eight people, it turned out, had come down with multiple sclerosis elsewhere and had retired to Duxbury as a good place to live out a chronic disease (Deacon, Alexander, Siedler and Kurland 1959).

Kurland (1994:S3) also gave a prime example of the importance of checking the validity of diagnoses even when there is a social explanation for an MS cluster. In the early 1950s he found that the highest MS death rate in all North America was reported for British Columbia. He thought it might be the result of people who developed the disease in eastern cities and moved to the milder climate of the Canadian west coast. Examining the death certificates, he found that the word "sclerosis" was written when "arterio-sclerosis" was the cause of death; "sclerosis" had been taken to signify "cerebral sclerosis," which was the World Health Organization term for MS at the time. This led to a quadrupling in the rate of MS deaths reported.

There have been clusters of MS reported in small towns (Galion, Ohio: see Turner 1986 and Henribourgh, Saskatchewan, Irvine 1989) and in factories (Stein et al. 1987). MS has also been among the diseases suffered by people dwelling near toxic-waste dumps (Love Canal). But a critical apparatus ensuring that the disease is actually MS must be in place before a cluster is verified.

Before the development of biochemical, electrophysical and imaging methods for determining multiple sclerosis in the living patient, the only way to be sure that someone had multiple sclerosis was to conduct an autopsy (which could hold surprises). This meant that the accuracy of mortality statistics depended on autopsies being matched with symptoms, and such matches were uncommon. "Autopsy is more likely to be carried out in rapid, difficult, or 'interesting' cases which constitute an unrepresentative fragment of the material. Thus Alter (1962) found that an autopsy was available in only one of 64 'probable' cases of multiple sclerosis in Negroes examined at the Neurological Institute in New York and this woman had died in the casualty department in an epileptic seizure" (Acheson 1972:7). E. D. Acheson casts doubt on the pre-test prevalence data as well, which are based on diagnoses that may not be borne out in autopsies made some time later (Pohlen 1942). Add to that the questionable procedures and possible results of racial bias in obtaining data on certain groups (e.g., African Americans in the United States, blacks in South Africa) and the practical question of case ascertainment becomes a matter of MS history. For all these reasons, the epidemiology formulated before unbiased diagnosis is an artifact. Some were aware of that and tried to prevent it from becoming a useless artifact.

Studying the rate of MS was best kept close to the source: prevalence studies in local areas by local practitioners had at least a chance of checking the validity of diagnoses. The establishment and promulgation of diagnostic standards more decisive than Charcot's triad helped identify cases as the same disease and thus enhanced the reliability of epidemiological studies. But the continued variation in names given to the disease signaled a variation in standards and international disparities in what should be counted as multiple sclerosis, which in turn confused any attempt to compare local prevalence studies to establish common factors. Etiologies multiplied and acquired their determined partisans.

Two significant types of information emerged: a study could determine the texture of case occurrence in an area as wide as Germany (Schaltenberg 1938) or Sweden (Müller 1949); or it could affirm the presence of a cluster of cases in a specific locale or set of similar locales. The accumulation of studies in the literature invited comparison both across time and from place to place. By the 1940s it had become possible to speculate on the relations between multiple sclerosis and the geography by interpreting earlier epidemiological studies in relation to each other and to the differences in terrain (Shatin 1944). Since multiple sclerosis had been identified as such on death certificates for several decades, mortality rates formed another body of epidemiological data ready for geographical reading (Limberg 1950).

A compendium of cluster studies, such as the 50-year span covered by T. H. Ingalls (1986), could then provide evidence for an etiology. Ingalls found that clustering of cases reported between 1934 and 1984 was consistent with a viral epidemiology. Whatever the findings of the pathologists, or their lack of findings, geography supported further investigation into the possibility of a viral cause.

Another benefit of the mass of prevalence studies was a refinement in record-keeping. Much more could be learned from epidemiology if details such as childhood infections or the condition of siblings were also noted. Many early studies were not as valuable as they might have been because the same data were not recorded for each case. A study of a factor might founder because the same piece of information measured according to the same standards was not available for a significant number of cases or by its nature could not be available. The trauma hypothesis, which had gathered anecdotal evidence since Charcot's time, was particularly difficult to assess epidemiologically. It was difficult to collect enough information about an MS patient's injuries to support or disprove the theory.

As in the epidemiology of other diseases, suspicions about causes encouraged single-factor surveys of known MS populations. How does multiple sclerosis prevalence correspond with concentrations of lead in the environment (Warren 1974)? Does relative pork consumption predict the likelihood of multiple sclerosis (Nanji and Narod 1986)?

Comprehensively collecting data on diagnosis has also led to multifactorial studies and the inclusion of multiple sclerosis risk factors among data routinely gathered from all patients or the elevation of items of data routinely collected from all patients to multiple sclerosis risk factors. In 1947 A. R. MacLean and colleagues at the Mayo Clinic in Rochester, Minnesota, presented a paper at a meeting of the Association for Research in Mental Nervous Diseases (in New York); they brought together data collected in Rochester over the previous two decades. The depth of the admission and followup records kept at the clinic allowed a model presentation of the prevalence and incidence of multiple sclerosis in a population better defined geographically and socially than in any previous study. The close historical relationship between the Mayo Clinic and the general population in Rochester made it more likely that those afflicted would come to the clinic and would return there over the course of their illness, reducing ascertainment problems at least by making them more visible.

Incidence is a measure of the number of cases of a disease diagnosed within a particular period of time. The MacLean paper found that prevalence in Rochester was double the generally expected rate (60 rather than 30 per 100,000) and that incidence remained steady over the period studied. Since there was no evidence of an MS epidemic in Rochester, it had to be suspected that MS was more common than previously believed and that lower reported rates meant faulty ascertainment.

The Mayo team also had the first substantial data on survival rates after diagnosis, which averaged 35 years, almost three times the average found in hospital-based studies. This implied that people going to hospitals were more advanced in their disease and that the clinic was likely to reach a larger number of people afflicted with multiple sclerosis earlier in their disease. The Mayo Clinic expanded its epidemiological purview of multiple sclerosis to include a number of factors that might be associated with the disease, attracting researchers and clinicians who both used and contributed to the growing body of data. In 1968 (Percy et al. 1968) a 60-year survey was published. By 1989 the spatial dimensions of the data drawing on the records of other health care institutions had expanded to include all of Olmstead County, Missouri. With the addition of sources from the years 1903 to 1915, when the Mayo Clinic was still part of St. Mary's Hosital, the time range was 80 years, in effect constituting a history of the appearance of multiple sclerosis in an American rural locale. The Rochester Project (Wynn et al. 1989) was a model for the delineated population study of chronic disease, both extensive and expensive, requiring precise standardized diagnosis and dedicated record-keeping over a long period of time.

The Rochester Project multiplied etiological factors rather than eliminated them: it did not prove a decisive test in favor of any one theory of multiple sclerosis origins. In having gained the ability to pursue a variety of factors through time, this type of epidemiology lost the comparative dimension of space, which increasingly seemed a key to the nature of multiple sclerosis.

Within the United States, at least, some of this deficiency in the data was made up by another type of information, collected from a nationwide body using a uniform system of clinical record-keeping: the Veterans' Administration studies of ex-servicemen during the late 1950s (Acheson 1972:25-26). This gender-biased survey discovered a north-to-south decreasing gradient when cases were distributed by place of birth. It also projected the finding that MS was more prevalent among African Americans than among Euro-Americans, though this was contradicted by other studies.

Physicians with European or American training working in colonies of the European nations did not take long to conclude that the disease was uncommon among native peoples of Africa, South Asia and Polynesia (e.g., 617 whites and 9 Maoris were admitted to New Zealand hospitals between 1950 and 1957; Acheson 1972:34). There appears to be a "racial predilection" for multiple sclerosis (Alter and Harshe 1975). McDonald (1993:885) even goes so far as to state, "No postmortem-proved case has yet been described in African blacks." The "postmortem-proved" component of that statement itself suggests that the state of information is not what it should be. In his critical review of African multiple sclerosis, C. M. Poser (1996) concludes that despite overestimations and misdiagnoses, MS has been demonstrated in native black Africans but is extremely rare and seems to grow more common with white admixture. This, in conjunction with a similar pattern found in the rest of the tropics, he takes to support a genetic world epidemiology of MS.

As enough information became available to permit tentative generalizations, a world geography of multiple sclerosis began to establish itself: the disease is much more likely to occur in the temperate zones and much less likely to occur in the tropics. McDonald adds that, "prevalence of the disease is lower in American blacks than in whites living in the same area" (McDonald 1993:885). One of the first questions that arises is whether this correspondence is centered on latitude alone or on genetic makeup.

The answer might come with the study of migration: if people from the zone of greatest susceptibility were much less likely to come down with multiple sclerosis after migrating to the tropics, then some aspect of latitude is the key factor. If, on the other hand, susceptibility among migrant populations remained the same as in the tropics, then a racial or a genetic factor is predominant in determining infection. Testing this conclusion requires comparable data for different groups in the same area, for blacks as well as whites. For a time, these data were embarrassingly absent.

There were two obvious migrations that would permit racial comparisons at the same latitude: of blacks to the north (mostly a forced migration) and of whites to the south (colonization). The United States began to yield up clinically uniform epidemiology including both blacks and whites in the same measures only with the veterans' surveys of the late 1950s, and even then there was not sufficient information for a racial comparison. F. Georgi and P. Hall (1960), as part of an assault on the "problematic" of multiple sclerosis, compared the Swiss prevalence rates with those obtained from Kenya. With the limited mortality records available, they concluded the disease is very uncommon among nonwhites. The lack of accurate records (no postmortem) of multiple sclerosis among Africans in Africa or in diaspora made and makes it difficult to compare rates internationally on both a racial and a latitude-climactic basis. The first migration studies, therefore, did not compare multiple sclerosis rates among whites with rates among blacks either in southern- or in northern-latitude countries. They compared rates among white migrants in Africa with rates among whites in the parent European countries because of the superior medical attention given whites. MS may be a "white man's burden" (Kurtzke 1983:90) in more ways than one.

Geoffrey Dean (1949), intending to study the relationship between multiple sclerosis incidence and the incidence of a disease in sheep (not a frivolous investigation), found that MS is relatively rare among whites in South Africa. However, he discovered a distinction within the white population: the Boers had a lower prevalence than those of British descent. Recognizing the disadvantages of using only mortality records, Dean undertook a more extensive and intensive survey (1967); checking diagnostic records and mortality notations, he confirmed the original Boer/British disparity in rates. Recent migrants of either group were developing multiple sclerosis at a rate comparable to that of their home regions; whereas both groups, even after a single generation, were showing a lower rate, the rate of the Boers was much lower than that of the British.

The migration studies substantiated both latitude and genetic conceptions of multiple sclerosis etiology. There was something about Dutch-Boer makeup that caused them to respond to the rate-reducing effects of latitude more positively than did the British, and there was something about latitude that reduced the rate in both populations. Israel was a test case in which a

European population, albeit diverse, migrated en masse to a lower latitude, where they had access to medical facilities comparable to those available to native-born Israelis ("with the possible exception of the Arabs"). The multiple sclerosis prevalence among the immigrants could be compared with the rate among Israelis. Though M. Alter's study (1960) did show a lower rate among the native-born, later studies (Leibowitz, Kahana and Alter 1969) with larger numbers of cases called this conclusion into doubt. The prevalence seemed to be about equal among immigrants and native-born.

Though it has become a cliché of MS epidemiology that prevalence decreases among immigrants from high prevalence to low prevalence zones (usually north to south) and increases among immigrants in the opposite direction, the amount of high-quality data actually available to support this conclusion is very limited. Large populations have not been relocated to different latitudes long enough within the era of more precise lifetime diagnosis for migration studies to have strong validity. And the statement that native peoples do not come down with multiple sclerosis seems an excuse for poor services. Perhaps the observation that age of migration decides prevalence is more supportable. It has been found that people migrating before puberty are likely to develop MS at the rate of their dwelling site, whereas those who migrated earlier keep to the rate at their latitude of origin. The Israeli (Alter, Leibowitz and Speer 1966) and South African (Kurtzke, Dean and Botha 1970) data support this conclusion, but Asian migrants to more southerly latitudes in North America do not show any change of rate (Detels, Brody and Edgar 1972). Multiple sclerosis continues to be rare among Asian migrants. This inspires the speculation that latitude change leads to prevalence change only in populations in which MS is relatively common.

Some of those countries with the longest history of multiple sclerosis epidemiology studies (Switzerland, Italy, France, former Soviet Union) show north-to-south prevalence gradients, but just as many (England, Germany, Sweden) do not. An examination of 200 prevalence studies completed between 1940 and 1980 outlines a north-to-south gradient in North America and most of Europe and a south-to-north gradient in Australia and New Zealand (Kurtzke and Kurland 1983). A north-to-south gradient in Japan is asserted on the basis of a very small number of cases and a definition of MS that includes conditions not included in the Euro-American category (Poser 1996).

A long history of studies also has uncovered nonlatitude-related variations in frequency of multiple sclerosis in the Scandinavian countries and in Switzerland. High rates inland and lower rates along the seacoast have been asserted and questioned for Norway: even in these medically sophisticated areas, there may be correlation between prevalence and the number of doctors responding to questionnaires (how much more so in countries with concentrated facilities?). One simple fact about epidemiology in the northern

European countries and Switzerland is that "the variation is between very and moderately common rather than between common and rare" (Acheson 1972:39). This, then, suggests that variations in rates in areas where MS is already rare may not be statistically significant and have no bearing on the study of etiology.

The history of multiple sclerosis epidemiology has always been a search for concentrations of cases that — in relation to some discernible environmental, social or infective factor — might reveal at least one possible precipitating cause. The data gathered in this search best fit what Kurtzke (1983:91) calls the "simple" or "prevalence" hypothesis of multiple sclerosis: "the cause of MS will be found where the clinical disease is common." Any instance of cases clustered together could be very revealing and provide guidance for analysis of existing data and a plan for further studies. Finding these revealing clusters might proceed by multiple sclerosis revealing itself in an actual epidemic or by researchers locating a factor that would then provide a correlation, which could also be indicated by an epidemic. History can be made to move as a sorting out of factors.

Multiple sclerosis history, both biological and cultural, has been a void because it has not provided an epidemic. The normal distribution of the disease — north and south, by race and so on — has been frustratingly normal: this is a disease for which 100 cases per 100,000 population is considered a high rate of prevalence; 500 per 100,000 would certainly constitute an epidemic, but such a level of infection has never been reported. The only MS epidemics seem to occur in very small populations. But improving diagnostic standards may yet demonstrate much higher "normal" prevalences and incidences.

An epidemic of nine clustered cases in Kenya (Adams 1989) leaves some doubts about the accuracy of the diagnosis but, if verified, might support a viral etiology. A point clustering of cases — three Olympic skiers (Heuga, Stier and Zimmerman) in the 1964 Innsbruck games — has not disclosed a more distinctive correlation than Olympic participation and the fact that all three skiers are from high-prevalence areas.

During the period after the occupation of the Faroe Islands by British troops from 1939 to 1945 there was a surge of MS where there had been none previously, at least according to J. F. Kurtzke and K. Hyllested (1975). By reviewing hospital records in the Faroes and Copenhagen (the islands are a Danish dependency), death certificates and disability compensation files and by interviewing family members, Kurtzke and Hyllested identified 107 possible cases of multiple sclerosis. Excluding some cases on the basis of uncertainty, outside origins or travel away from the islands, they arrived at a total of 32 cases without symptoms before 1940, 16 of whom suffered their onset between 1942 and 1950. In all, there were three epidemics between 1943 and 1973. This appeared to demonstrate that MS is an infectious and transmissible disease brought to the previously isolated Faroes by the occupying troops and possibly spread by the troops themselves.

In a special issue of the journal *Neuroepidemiology* devoted to the Faroes epidemic, C. M. Poser et al. (1988) criticized the conclusion that there had been an epidemic. Insisting that 10 of the excluded cases be added to the 32, they showed that at least 2 of the cases had their onset before the British troops ever arrived and that only 15 of the 42 were in the "vulnerable" five-to-fourteen-year-old age range during the occupation. The impression that there was an epidemic was due, according to the Poser team, to inadequate case ascertainment before the arrival of the British and to the fact that the Faroes probably share a high prevalence with other North Sea countries. "The theory of transmission is unconvincing and the characteristics of the putative agent unrealistic. The extremely high incidence of disease, which has statistical significance, is based on a very small number of cases in a very small population" (Poser et al. 1988:168).

Kurtzke and Hyllested's rebuttal of Poser and his colleagues' criticism was included in the same issue of *Neuroepidemiology* (1988:190-227). It consists largely of a case-by-case reclaiming of support for a sequence of epidemics on the islands. But Geoffrey Dean, in the editorial leading the edition, judges the epidemic "not proven." Multiple sclerosis did not occur as an epidemic among many other island populations visited by Europeans. Though an infective agent has long been theorized, there still is no evidence of an agent in tissues. Accepting that there may have been an increase in the number of cases of multiple sclerosis on the Faroes if not an epidemic, Poser and his team point out the great stress visited on the islanders by the war, the heavy casualties, the building of new roads reducing social isolation, changes in diet and even an epidemic of canine distemper (a disease caused by a virus resembling the virus that causes measles in humans). There were many other risk factors at work other than human-to-human infection.

The epidemiology of MS continues to be subject more to the advance of Western medicine into remote parts of the world than to any other factor. Supposed epidemics on the Shetland and Orkney Islands (Poskanzer et al. 1980), even less verifiable than the Faroes epidemic, also attended the commercial development of the islands. Multiple sclerosis epidemiology is the history of human movements, of changes in the standard of medical records and diagnostic procedures. Only secondarily is it a record of MS itself. Before World War II, the Faroes were an obscure set of islands in Danish possession. Immigration and emigration had taken place before the war, but they intensified during and after, increasing the flow of information or of infection, however you choose to view it. Rather than reading the history from the epidemiology, we might want to read the epidemiology from the history. We might be able to see more clearly how historical events like migrations provide and have provided a motive to form epidemiologies of MS.

11

From Infection to Autoimmunity

Toward the end of 1921, the Association for Research in Nervous and Mental Disease held a meeting in New York City predominantly devoted to multiple sclerosis. The keynote paper was presented by the British neurologist Sir James Purves-Stewart, head of neurology for the Allied Expeditionary Forces, who spoke on war trauma. But he also was very interested in MS.

In their article "General Symptomatology and Differential Diagnosis of Multiple Sclerosis," which headed off the issue of *Archives of Neurology and Psychiatry* devoted to the meeting, Bernard Sachs and E. D. Friedman (1922) made a historical distinction. The earlier studies of MS concentrated on MS in its later stages of pathology and were dedicated primarily to gathering histological evidence. The newer studies were focusing on the early stages of MS pathology and on the process of the disease rather than its outcomes. The European students of MS had fostered a wealth of categorically opposed theories of MS pathology, some arguing that it is rare, others that it is common, some that it is exogenous (caused by an outside agent) and infectious (syphilitic) or postinfectious (Marie's encephalomyelitis), some that it is endogenous (caused by internal processes) and degenerative, others that is endogenous and toxic. Declaring it to be "one of the few nonsyphilitic diseases of the central nervous system," Sachs and Friedman broke with explicit and implicit attempts to explain MS in terms of underlying venereal disease while allowing an opening for the possibility of other exogenous agents. The "fresh start" that they sought included a rejection of the background of venereology in medicine of the central nervous system. But they apparently remained open to nonsyphilitic spirochetes. Sachs, who had compiled a list of the chief symptoms of MS in 1898, included his own list among those symptoms now to be put aside in favor of a revised symptomatology.

In 1924 the Société Neurologique de Paris held its fifth meeting since the war, and the subject was *sclérose en plaques*, with comprehensive reports published in *Revue Neurologique* (Veraguth and Guillain 1925) and with a number of papers on the histology, symptomatology and psychiatry of MS. German participants joined the French and Dutch, but there were few British or Americans delivering papers. The French defended the Charcotian account of symptoms, which did include an investigation of the earlier stages, and the diagnostic preeminence of the triad, but they confessed, as had the Americans in 1922, that the causes and the immediate development of the disease were poorly understood while putting forward various theories. The multiplicity of causes and the similarities between MS and many other diseases motivated Veraguth to call it one of the great enigmas of neurology. There still was no effective treatment.

Smith Ely Jelliffe, who had been studying MS in his patients since the turn of the century, repeated Veraguth's remark in his textbook on diseases of the central nervous system, a book he coauthored with the psychiatrist William Alanson White in 1935. Jelliffe and White included a brief account of the history of MS diagnosis at the beginning of the section on "multiple sclerosis syndromes" (Jelliffe and White 1935:590). They recognized that MS patients had long been grouped under other conditions and that it was only with the visual images of the lesions shown by Carswell and Cruveilhier (in line drawings) and the symptomatologies of Frerichs, Valentiner, Vulpian, Ordenstein and Charcot that a disease entity took shape. They then summarized (with citations) the conclusions arising from the research that had proceeded both in Europe and in the United States since the end of the war.

> More recent research tends to show that strict nosological boundaries are extremely difficult to draw between closely related syndromes. The view that differing kinds of toxi-infectious noxae can bring about more or less disseminated encephalomyelitic pictures is gaining ground. There are still facts which maintain, in part, the older conceptions of a chronic degenerative vascular process while at the same time there is increasing evidence that a more or less acute infectious process brings about the greater number of cases. The present description follows the conception that there is a primary endogenous picture of unknown etiology with fairly uniform pathology, and a number of secondary forms of exogenous multiform etiology and diverse pathologies. The symptoms are largely matters of localization.

The announced turn from a static pathology of existing MS to an examination of the degeneration in process had yielded significant new evidence in the years between the New York meeting and the publication of Jelliffe and White's text. The American and European research during the interval underwrote the statement that MS is primarily endogenous (not caused by an invading agent). The process of tissue damage within the body was unknown, whereas the symptoms could be understood from the location of the plaques. The spine was the original locus of MS, but the American studies now centered around the brain, territory Charcot had avoided.

Experimentation on living animals and not the study of dead human tissue led to these conclusions. The conditions believed to induce degeneration had to be replicated in living tissue. There could be no experimentation on human subjects and no removal of living human tissue for test purposes. Animals had been used in nerve mapping and physiology experiments from early times but only peripherally in MS research until the postwar period. The tradition of Pinel, Bichat and Cruveilhier emphasized the uniqueness of human tissues and rejected animal experiments. The clinical pathology method excluded animal studies in favor of following human cases through to postmortem ("You will find no dog clinic in my laboratories," Charcot told the visiting German neurologist Hirt). But the postwar Great Britain and United States had a shortage of human pathology specimens, and the animal experiments had revealed the fundamental identity of all mammalian nerve tissue. Jelliffe and White were able to make their circumspect summation because of experiments on rabbits, dogs, cats and rats deliberately subjected to toxins and circumstances that the postmortem study of human nerve matter suggested might bring about multiple sclerosis. The newly dynamic multiple sclerosis research could gain access to the process itself only by trying to bring it about and then watch it unfold in animal bodies.

A proposition immediately subject to experimentation was that MS, like many other mysterious conditions, might be caused by an invasive bacterium or microorganism. The knowledge that specific microbes always caused malaria or plague suggested that any disease of unknown etiology might be understood in the same way.

A spirochete (Treponema) pertenue was already known to cause gonorrhea. After Erich Hoffmann and Fritz Schaudinn discovered (1905) spirochete (Treponema) pallidum as the pathogen of syphilis, there were attempts to find a spirochete at the root of MS.

Charles L. Dana of the Cornell Medical College stated at the 1921 New York meeting that he "assumed ... some variety of spirochaetae" to be at the bottom of MS (1922:43). Dana was the author of the standard neurology text in America, *Text-book of Nervous Diseases* (1892 and many editions thereafter), in which he favored an infectious theory of disseminated sclerosis. The European research was also the context of Sachs and Friedman's statement that MS was the commonest "non-syphilitic" disease of the central nervous system: it still might be caused by a nonsyphilitic spirochete, an abundance of which live on human skin and in the mouth. Dana was basing his assumption on work by German microbiologists, who in 1917–18 claimed to have induced experimental disseminated sclerosis in animals. Peter Kuhn and Gabriel Steiner injected guinea pigs and rabbits with spinal fluid and blood of MS patients, causing them to become paralyzed, then injected the blood of the paralyzed animals into healthy animals, inducing paralysis through four passages in guinea pigs and two in rabbits (in obedience to Koch's rules for verifying bacterial presence). They compared the resultant symptoms and pathology with a leptospira (also a spirochete) infection and named the agent *Spirochaeta argentinensis*. But spirochetes are notoriously difficult to discern under the microscope: the one that causes syphilis had been identified (by Hoffmann and Schaudinn) only in 1905. And they were impossible to culture outside living bodies. The evidence for the MS spirochete remained experimental.

D. K. Adams (1921), while agreeing that the great weight of clinical evidence is against a syphilitic basis for MS, tells of his own experiments diagnosing MS with the Lange gold test of cerebrospinal fluid (spirochete reactive) and then successfully treating patients with anti-spirochete ("modern anti-specific") compounds. Though Adams's reported cases both were men, a London neurologist's use of his treatment on a woman is probably what inspired Barbellion to believe that a cure for his disease was becoming available (October 5, 1918). The development of anti-spirochete drugs (Ehrlich's salvarsan) spurred efforts to find what other diseases were caused by these elusive organisms.

At the 1921 New York meeting, Oscar Teague reported the "practically negative" results of his own attempts to replicate the European tests and cited several other unsuccessful attempts to induce infections in animals with MS patient bodily fluids. The Commission of the Association for Research into Mental and Nervous Diseases acknowledged the negative result and counseled "a cautious appreciation of the finding of micro-organism in this disease" (Teague 1922:208).

Neurosyphilis symptoms are so similar to those of MS that it is difficult to discard the belief that MS can be treated as a spirochete-caused disease. The psychiatrist Julius Wagner-Jauregg, following on the earlier discovery that fever reduces mental symptoms, used malaria to treat asylum patients afflicted with general paresis of the insane, generally a syphilitic condition. Wagner-Jauregg won the 1927 Nobel prize in medicine and physiology for his innovation, which during its heyday was applied to a variety of other diseases thought to be caused by spirochetes, including MS.

As late as 1952 Gabriel Steiner, one of the 1918 researchers, was finding spirochetes, which he called *Spirochaeta myelophthora*, in specimens of acute MS plaques he had meticulously prepared and stained. In the years between those studies and the 1950s, Steiner had a career as a neuroanatomist. Steiner defended his findings in a series of papers in English-language medical journals and in a comprehensive German text (Steiner 1962). The *New York Times* reported on June 8, 1957, that R. Ichelson had isolated "*Spirochaeta myelophthora*," the microorganism that causes MS. Ichelson claimed to have perfected a test for MS. In December of the same year she announced that St. Luke's Children's Medical Center in Philadelphia was adopting it. The renewed search for a spirochete at the base of MS may have been driven by the availability of penicillin and other antibiotics known to be effective against syphilis and gonorrhea. Penicillin in sufficiently intense doses always overcomes syphilis, but it has no direct effect on MS.

C. E. Lumsden (1958:753), commenting on Steiner's and other claims of spirochetes in MS material, shows photomicrographs of spirochete-like formations in MS plaques. The distinctive shape of spirochetes can be mimicked in the tissue peculiarities of MS lesions where no organisms at all are present. The success in isolating the syphilis spirochete at the beginning of the century continued to serve as a model for finding a spirochete culprit within MS.

The zoological genus *Spirochete* was renamed *Treponema* and Spirochetae was left as the name of the order in which Treponematae is a family and *Treponema* a genus. Spirochetes became a much broader category that includes other spiral bacteria, the Borreliae that cause Lyme disease and the Leptospirae that cause Fort Bragg fever, seven-day fever and others. Lyme disease, first attributed to the spirochete *Borrelia burgdorferi* in 1981, is easily mistaken symptomatically for MS (Barbour 1996:198–99). That a disease with such MS-like symptoms is caused by a spirochete reinforces the long-held idea of spirochete involvement in MS and keeps alive a shadow of the old syphilis explanation.

Steiner's *Spirochaeta myelophthora* was an anachronism looking back to the nomenclature of his earlier work in Germany. Even as Americans broke away from European MS studies, Steiner was able to implant the image of an MS spirochete. He won followers, like Ichelson, who tried to introduce tests and therapies based on spirochetical MS, against opposition from physicians and researchers who did not accept the proffered evidence. Other researchers, though not accepting or even recognizing the Steiner tradition, discovered their own spirochetes.

This is because spirochetes have been shown to be so versatile in their infectivity. The same *Treponema pertenue* that causes syphilis also causes bejel, a nonsyphilitic skin disease of wide distribution in the Middle East and Northern Africa. It has not been possible to differentiate the spirochetes causing the two diseases even on the genetic level. It therefore seems possible that the seemingly harmless spirochetes living in and on the human body have infectious strains and tempers. D. Gay and G. Dick (1986) argued in favor of an oral spirochete infection behind MS, and V. Marshall (1988) postulated a systemic spirochete infection as an explanation for the diverse effects of MS.

In 1996 Dr. Luther Lindner of Texas A&M University had an Internet site promoting blood tests to determine the presence of "the MS organism," the same *Spirochaeta myelophthora* that Steiner and Ichelson described, only

Lindner calls them "spirochete-like bacteria." Lindner's tests are to help judge which antibiotics are best to treat the patient's MS. "Why not just dose up the patient with antibiotics and hope for the best? Actually this is being widely done, with some success. The problem is that there may be little or no guidance as to when to stop." Lindner's test lab and a few others he names can provide that guidance. Spirochetes are here to stay.

The search for infectious microbial agents initiating some aspect of the MS process diversified with the discovery of new types of microbes. Viruses, first ascertained in the work of Pasteur's laboratory on rabies, were thought to be bacterial toxins that managed accidentally to pass through filters fine enough to eliminate bacteria. The Latin word "virus" (poison) was originally used to connote any unknown toxin but after the turn of the century came to be used for a substance that could pass through a fine filter yet seemed to be able to proliferate in living bodies in a way that an inorganic poison could not.

The name *filterable virus* was used until the middle of the century to distinguish this type of virus from other toxins, which could be filtered out. Diphtheria, tetanus and other bacteria were found in the late nineteenth century to cause their worst damage through a poison that passes through filters that exclude the bacteria themselves. Distinguishing inert bacterial viruses from other, proliferative viruses was one of the many practical tasks of definition. Viruses were not visible under the microscope, nor could they be detected by any of the blood serum tests applied to bacteria. The only way to determine the presence of a virus was to inject a filtered body fluid into a subject animal and observe the symptoms that develop. Like the bacteriological studies, the search for the MS virus gave impetus to animal experimentation in MS research.

In 1911–12 the English researcher W. E. Bullock injected cerebrospinal fluid from MS patients subcutaneously into domestic rabbits and within 19 to 22 days saw four out of five of the animals become paralyzed in the hindquarters (Bullock 1913). A microscope examination of spinal cord sections treated with the myelin stain developed by Marchi (1884) showed that the myelin sheathing had stained black, which was taken to indicate infiltration by an organic agent, though MS in humans did not stain like this. Since the human cerebrospinal fluid had been filtered and no new bacteria were microscopically visible, Bullock believed that a virus must be at work. This conclusion was encouraged by her inability to produce the same results when trying to infect captive wild rabbits, who may have been resistant to viruses through prior exposure. She did not proceed with the next step of the experiment: infect other rabbits with cerebrospinal fluid of presumably infected rabbits. Other researchers in Germany did try this, with guinea pigs and rabbits, but they saw the results as evidence of a spirochete. Researchers in France in 1918 confirmed these findings, but in 1921 researchers in Germany and Sweden could not replicate Bullock's findings (Teague 1922). Friedman and Sachs, in their 1922 article, relegated an exogenous (viral or bacterial) etiology to secondary status, but they did not rule it out.

When Bullock resumed her work under her married name, W. E. Gye, she was interested in testing for the viral etiology of malignant cancers (Gye 1925). Though only 17 of the 129 rabbits she injected developed paralysis, she was content to call this a confirmation of her earlier research and to identify a viral agent. Whereas Gye used primarily a fluid culture medium, her colleague J. E. Barnard turned to the agar slip method developed by Paul Ehrlich and cultured several animal and human cancer viruses. He published the photomicrographs and diagrams, claiming they showed virus colonies (Barnard 1925).

Gye's and Barnard's work extrapolated from the bacteria-like infectiousness of filterable viruses to the idea that if cultured properly, viruses — like bacteria — would produce colonies with specific visible and microscopic characteristics. This method proposed to overcome the frustrating physical invisibility of viruses by causing them to multiply up to the level of visibility.

This logic and method were so appealing that Kathleen Chevassut and Sir James Purves-Stewart (the same Purves-Stewart who had delivered the keynote address at the 1921 New York meeting) applied it to the hypothetical MS virus. As Chevassut and Purves-Stewart reported in papers published in *The Lancet* (1930), following Gye's and Barnard's methods they were able to generate virus colonies similar in appearance to Barnard's cancer virus colonies. Chevassut also was able to detect acid formation in dextrose broth to which MS patient blood serum had been added, the acid likely to explain the eating away of myelin (lipolysis) that preceded MS plaque formation. In the *British Medical Journal* Purves-Stewart (1930) even declared that he had obtained a vaccine for the treatment of disseminated encephalomyelitis. Using the model of smallpox vaccines, he had isolated the active agent of cerebral myelin degeneration and was able to administer it to likely victims in order to build a resistance to infection.

Like many explanations and promised cures before and since, this one was an illusion of human logic imposed on a far subtler biology. Arthur Weil of the Institute of Neurology at the Northwestern University Medical School visited Purves-Stewart and Chevassut's laboratory at Westminster Hospital in London. Weil (1931) described the equipment and culture procedures and the resultant agar culture slips showing spheres, many with a small granule attached. But the same colonies appeared when the slips were not incubated, and the same culture also could be made from the serum of patients with hyperthyroidism or pulmonary tuberculosis. This pattern of spheres and granules results when substances like those used in the cultures are subject to the same temperatures and mixing conditions: the appearance is the result of colloidal chemistry and is not due to a virus in the MS patients' spinal fluid. Weil also commented on the possibility that an acid "lipolytic ferment" in the spinal fluid or blood of MS patients might be causing the myelin to degenerate. His own experiments discounted this possibility as well.

Jelliffe and White's 1935 declaration that MS originated within the patient arose from the sometimes blatant failures to demonstrate a bacterial or viral MS agent. None of this prevented experimenters from carrying out further projects testing the infectiousness of human MS body fluids in animals or in cultures. An exogenous etiology of MS would hold against the older endogenous view that emphasized heredity and familial causes. Colin Talley (1995:40) believes that the epidemiological identity of MS as a disease endogenous to people of the "white races" may have delayed research into bacterial and viral agents (exogenous, which might infect anyone) until the 1910s. Possibly, the persistent search for single outside agents at the root of MS leads to avoiding a strictly hereditary, even racial idea of the disease. As a study of MS epidemiology shows, however, more medical attention may be the only reason MS seems confined to whites.

Jelliffe and White remained open to the possibility of many exogenous etiologies operating at the same time as endogenous ones, but they point to a primary acute process that actually brings about the damage, however it is precipitated. Many infectious and poisonous agents had been indicted. It might even turn out that a virus was among them. Chevassut and Purves-Stewart had been trying to prove that a virus was the primary pathological factor, that its action damaged the myelin. Other researches attempted to ascertain what could damage myelin in a way that resembled the damage seen in MS.

Experiments had to be planned to reveal the dynamic pathology of the disease and not just to demonstrate changes induced in inert tissue samples. Diseases known to cause an acute destruction of myelin might not cause sclerotic patches to form. During the late nineteenth century some researchers studying differential diagnosis (Leyden) believed that multiple sclerosis strictly as plaque formation was a chronic expression of acute myelopathies caused by a microbe, while others (Westphal) held that the acute disease and the sclerotic process were different. The lack of cases of acute myelopathy shown at autopsy made it impossible to establish which of these alternatives was true. Patients with what appeared to be acute multiple sclerosis either recovered or died very quickly. In either event, there was no disclosure of the relationship between acute multiple sclerosis and the eventual formation of plaques, the hallmark of MS. Those who did have MS symptoms in life and plaques at autopsy may or may not have had an acute episode earlier. By the 1920s there were not yet enough cases on record to decide that plaques of chronic MS always formed after an acute encephalomyelitis. Animals would provide a laboratory in which acute attacks could be induced and the aftermath followed to learn if the characteristic cerebral picture of MS emerged to any degree.

At the American Medical Association meeting in Philadelphia on June 11, 1931, Tracy Putnam, John B. McKenna and L. Raymond Morrison (1931) read a summary of their experiments inducing experimental animal encephalopathies. Putnam was a career neurologist. His uncle, James Jackson Putnam, first professor of neurology at Harvard, had made one of the early epidemiological studies of the spinal sclerosis (1897); the elder Putnam's obituary was included in the 1922 *Archives of Neurology and Psychiatry* issue that reported the New York meeting. Putnam himself had a diverse international training in neuroanatomy and diagnosis. Barends Brouwer, who theorized that the array of MS symptoms was due to evolutionary age of nervous system components, was one of Putnam's mentors.

For Putnam and his co-workers, the acute-chronic MS problem resolved into two main questions: whether acute disseminated encephalomyelitis is an infectious disease and whether acute demyelination "may or must always lead to a sclerotic patch if the subject survives." In humans and animals a number of diseases had been identified in which there was a swift demyelination usually in the vicinity of blood vessels, preservation of the axon cylinders and infiltration of glial cells, basically the Charcotian cellular pathology, together with a symptom set that did not allow clear differentiation among diseases. The experimenters attempted to induce the pathology in living animals.

Following the methods of previous researchers, Putnam and collaborators inoculated dogs with tetanus toxin, subjected both dogs and cats to pure carbon monoxide and induced cerebral thromboses by injecting dogs and cats with a cod liver oil emulsion. All three techniques caused permanent myelin loss in the animals' brains and a progressive infiltration of glial cells at the site of the demyelination: "all three resemble closely the 'early' plaques of multiple sclerosis." In the carbon monoxide and cod liver oil thrombotic lesions, obstruction of the blood vessels seemed to play a part in formation, as lesions also in those caused by tetanus toxin. This was the rapid onset of multiple sclerosis symptoms that presumably accompanied the rapid destruction of myelin. Rapid action could be observed experimentally; slow degeneration over a period of years might just be the slower form of the same process or the slow exposure of symptoms.

Putnam and his colleagues were experimenting with different potential agents: a bacterial toxin, an airborne asphyxiant and a vascular thrombotic. This choice was based on the assumption that the vascular lesions discovered in humans who had died from carbon monoxide poisoning or tetanus resembled those of MS. George Hassin, listening to the presentation of the paper in 1931 (and seeing the photomicrographs of tissue samples), agreed that MS is caused by a toxin rather than an infection. Presenting in his study of the pathogenesis of MS at the 1922 meeting, Hassin had declared in favor of the noninfectious, toxic origins of MS lesions. But he did not accept that the lesions Putnam and colleagues had produced resembled even the "early" plaques of MS. MS damage does not occur naturally in dogs, he declared (inaccurately, as it turned out). "The patches produced experimentally probably looked like those seen in multiple sclerosis, but when one compares the early and late plaques of human multiple sclerosis with those demonstrated by Dr. Putnam, one may see that they are not the same" (Putnam, McKenna and Morrison 1931:1595). Hassin added that cases of encephalitis in humans also do not resemble MS pathologically. In MS, nerve destruction is followed by massive glial reaction, whereas in encephalitis (and in Putnam's experiments) all the effects take place simultaneously. Hassin maintained that Putnam did not successfully produce a model of MS in his animal subjects because he did not reproduce the sequence of events in MS. Putnam, in response, maintained that the later lesions in his subjects examined a year after exposure did resemble genuine MS lesions. The disagreement hinged on the macroscopic and microscopic resemblance of the experimental animal patches to human MS patches.

None of those present questioned the vascular basis of lesion formation. Whatever caused the damage must have entered the area through the cerebral arteries, and it must have been something deliverable by or through the vascular system. The pattern of destruction was common to several organic and inorganic agents. The experimental encephalopathy verified that multiple secondary etiologies could impinge on a single primary one, a localized toxification of blood flow. This certainly served a vascular primary degeneration. The complexity of MS might be numerous external and unrelated causes, several even at work on the same patient, leading to a single localized nerve degeneration.

That Putnam could not produce experimental MS, only an experimental encephalopathy that did not strongly resemble MS microscopically, supported the continued distinction between acute and chronic demyelinating diseases. They were not all versions of the same disease that ended as MS with plaques. This criticism of Putnam's study was sustained in other animal studies: true chronic MS could not be induced or observed in animals.

Putnam, McKenna and J. Evans (1932) boldly claimed they had induced "experimental multiple sclerosis" in dogs' brains by injecting them with tetanus toxin. The emphasis remained on the myelin destruction because it was the basis of so many other diseases that did not include plaque formation. Putnam's demonstrations purported to show that experimental encephalomyelitis was a basic stage that could lead to experimental multiple sclerosis. He was at pains to show that both sclerotic plaques and "encephalitis" were the productions of blood vessel blockage. Charcot had suggested embolism as a cause of MS, and in 1882 Ribbert had specified tiny blood thrombi in the capillaries as the immediate source of the plaques. In many other experiments and papers on into the 1940s, Putnam maintained that his artificially produced plaques were the same as MS plaques, that myelin decay preceded plaque formation and was itself a consequence of vascular obstruction. When the newly

founded National Multiple Sclerosis Society asked him to head the committee writing a manual for diagnosing physicians (Putnam et al. 1947), this is
the version of MS he set out in the face of other competing views, including
some that had arisen from his own research.

In a classification of demyelinating disease processes (Ferraro 1937), acute
disseminated encephalomyelitis arising spontaneously was distinguished pathologically from acute disseminated encephalomyelitis following acute infections
(measles, chicken pox, smallpox and vaccinations against smallpox). Disseminated sclerosis and diffuse sclerosis were distinguished from each other and
from the acute types, as was disseminated myelitis with optic neuritis. This
classification coalesced a number of the clinical entities that had been distinguished from each other earlier in the century, but it took the position that
there is an acute disseminated sclerosis distinct from acute disseminated
encephalomyelitis (see chart in Russell 1940:470). This was the technical
response to the failure to show that acute encephalomyelitis and chronic MS
are the same disease process.

That failure was also a failure of animal experiments specifically to model
human MS, which in turn led to the conclusion that the animals used were
not similar enough to humans to show the same effects that humans would
in response to vascular toxins. P. F. A. Hoefer, T. J. Putnam and M. G. Gray
(1938) cautiously referred to the experimental "encephalitis" they produced in
animals by injecting them with coagulants. Between the first study of 1931 and
1938, Putnam himself had published six more "Studies in Multiple Sclerosis"
in various journals, experimentally testing the vascular obstruction hypothesis through animal experiments. Though his experiments asserted a new vascular hypothesis of MS — that it was due to a blockage or thrombosis the
vessels causing local inflammation — he was not able to provide an animal
model of MS itself but only of acute disseminated encephalitis. MS remained
out of the experimenter's reach.

T. M. Rivers, D. H. Sprunt and G. P. Berry (1935) injected vaccine (smallpox) virus into the brains (cisterna magna) of rhesus monkeys and found no
evidence that the virus could produce an acute disseminated encephalomyelitis
with perivascular demyelination. When they gave intramuscular injections of
rabbit brain, however, they did find inflammation and demyelination of the
central nervous system resulting in two of the eight monkeys. This was another
demonstration that an infectious agent, a virus, was not causing one grade of
damage typical of MS-like diseases, but now there was a finding that brain
tissue from another animal could produce this damage in a few cases. These
experiments were based on the evidence building, since the first use of vaccines, that the vaccine medium, rabbit or rodent brain tissue, could at times
spur allergic damage to myelin.

In another set of experiments with monkeys performed around the same
time, Rivers and F. F. Schwentker (1935) followed a line of reasoning that led

away from the infection-inflammation debate. "The repeated intramuscular injections of aqueous emulsions and alcohol-ether extracts of sterile normal rabbit brains in some manner produced pathological changes accompanied by myelin destruction in the brains of 7 of 8 monkeys (*Macacus rhesus*). Eight control monkeys remained well. Cultures from the involved brains remained sterile, and no transmissible agent was demonstrated by means of intercerebral inoculations of emulsions of bits of the brains into monkeys, rabbits, guinea pigs, and white mice." The lesions they had induced in monkeys did not resemble the spontaneous lesions others had observed, but the lesions had a character that would lead them to suspect an infectious agent. Neither stains, cultures nor injecting experimental animals with brain emulsions gave any evidence of an infectious agent. Unable to maintain a large colony of monkeys to test all the possible variants, Rivers and Schwentker gave multiple injections to the same set of eight. They had tried to eliminate any possibility of an infection present in the samples they used, but they were not entirely sure they had. Nonetheless, it seemed to them that they had induced demyelination and other pathological changes (though no plaque formation) with sterile extracts that did not have the texture of thrombotics. The monkeys' demyelination was occurring in reaction to something in the rabbit brain.

In the Pasteur series of treatments administered to people possibly infected with rabies, rabbit brain serves as the medium for progressively more concentrated doses of the virus. About one patient in four thousand actually becomes paralyzed and is shown to have suffered demyelination. The rabbit brain alone appeared to cause demyelination in Rivers and Schwentker's experiments; they wondered if the same might be true in these human reactions to the Pasteur vaccine. But they did not have enough monkeys to try the necessary tests.

They were left with a basis for speculation and further experiment. Rabbit brain free from infectious agents had of its own accord induced encephalomyelitis in experimental subjects of another species. The same pair of experimenters (Schwentker and Rivers 1938) tried injecting monkeys with rabbit brain tissue that had been subjected to smallpox virus and then filtered free of the virus itself. They found that the monkeys showed the same demyelinating reaction and, further, that an extract from the reacting monkey brain tissue reacted to unaffected monkey brains. Following viral attack, the brain tissue generated a substance that caused it to respond as if identical tissue were foreign.

According to A. Ferraro and G. A. Jervis (1940:208), these experiments "proved that homologous brain altered by autolysis (breakdown) or by infection with vaccine virus becomes antigenic and is then capable of inducing the production of antibodies specific for brain tissue." They were using the language of immunology, antigens and antibodies, to describe the reactions obtained when infectious agents were eliminated from the brain tissue injected. This way of describing certain inflammatory reactions arose from studies of induced immunity to infectious disease (Behring and Kitasato 1890). It was believed that living systems produced specific antibodies in reaction to specific antigens, that tetanus antibodies were created in the encounter of bodily fluids with tetanus bacilli. The presence of antibodies could serve as the basis for chemical tests of the microbes' presence and for prevention and therapy, since antibodies could be transferred from someone infected with the microbe to someone who had not encountered it or was not producing adequate antibodies. Ferraro and Jervis's experiments led them to the conclusion that brain tissue itself could be transformed into an antigen by infection or degeneration and could stimulate the production of anti-brain tissue antibodies in living brain tissue.

Ferraro and Jervis had performed a version of Rivers's experiments. They inoculated seven monkeys with sterile rabbit brain extract over periods varying from four to thirteen months. The result was disseminated perivascular lesions "characterized by destruction of myelin and accumulations of fatty granular cells." There were also large areas of partial demyelination that showed no relation to blood vessels.

They compared this condition to the encephalomyelitis that sometimes developed in recipients of rabies vaccine. Indeed a similar pathology had been noticed by this time in reaction to other vaccines and blood serums (Winkelman and Gotten 1935). The foreign tissue used as the vaccine medium was causing the demyelination. In the discussion that followed the presentation of Ferraro and Jervis's paper, Dr. Ben Balser of New York told of experimentally inducing symptoms and a pathology strongly resembling disseminated sclerosis in a monkey on injection of a sterilized human brain extract. But the "accumulations of fat" (myelin breakdown products) on the spinal column and in the brain of the monkey were not concentrated around the blood vessels. In response, Jervis said that he and Ferraro had also seen fatty masses away from the vessels and that he considered the "problem of the formation of brain-specific antibodies" important enough to warrant further experiments.

These experiments already had been conducted, but now the ability to exclude viruses as well as bacteria from the injected extracts made findings more secure. Experimenters became more positive that the lesions they were producing in experimental animals and comparing with demyelination in humans were the result of a reaction by the brain tissues themselves. Several physiological models were called into service to describe this. L. M. Davidoff, B. C. Seegal and D. Seegal (1932) described "the Arthus phenomenon" in rabbit brains. This phenomenon was a localized inflammatory reaction that its discoverer, the French physiologist Maurice Arthus, observed at the site of tuberculin and other inoculations. A substance already existing in the tissue reacted chemically with the introduced substance. The gist of the Arthus reaction, however, was that the localized inflammation was far worse the second time the same substance was injected in the same place. The first injection had caused a substance (antibodies) to develop, which reacted to a substance (antigen) introduced with the injection. A similar phenomenon was detected in other bodily systems, for instance in the interactions of blood tabulated during wartime transfusion attempts. Davidoff, Seegal and Seegal caused an Arthus reaction in rabbit brains and compared the resulting lesions to demyelination in the human brain.

Performing the same kind of experiment with rhesus monkeys, N. Kopeloff, Davidoff and L. Kopeloff (1936) referred to the reaction as "anaphylaxis," a term from studies of injection site reactions to vaccines. They brought about general systemic anaphylaxis in the monkeys, sending the monkeys into a state of shock. They surveyed the cerebral lesions that resulted. This experimental anaphylaxis added the further component a localized antibody reaction in the brain to a generally administered antigen. The antibodies that had been formed in the wake of earlier injections of the same substance were brain-specific to the antigen. The brain could develop demyelination in response to a particular substance that might not cause reactions in other tissues or organs.

From Rivers's research in the early 1930s, the factors surrounding demyelination had been progressively narrowed down in experiments performed by a group of researchers small enough and in close enough contact for their conclusions to be progressive. Jervis and Ferraro joined Kopeloff and Kopeloff (1941) of the anaphylactic experiments to pool specimens and conclusions for a general study of the neuropathology of "experimental anaphylaxis" in monkeys. They confirmed that demyelination typically results from a systemic anaphylaxis. Jervis (1943) by himself performed experiments that epitomized all the findings in these series. He injected an aqueous extract of guinea pig kidney into rabbits, obtained the reactive portions (antibodies) from the rabbits' blood and injected them into the carotid artery of rabbits, leading once again to cerebral demyelination. No contaminating bacteria or virus seemed to be at work: the rabbit antibodies entered the circulatory system via the neck artery and did their damage in the brain. The damage was not simply a localized inflammation caused by injection of offensive substances directly into the brain, nor was it solely the result of thrombotic blockage of the cerebral blood vessels. The presence of an antibody in blood circulating close to the brain would lead to demyelination

The word *allergy*, an older and more general term than *anaphylaxis*, was used in connection with MS (F. Kennedy 1938; Baer and Sulzberger 1939), mainly to show the resemblance of allergic reactions in other parts of the body to cerebral damage caused by the same substances. A review of the literature led Ferraro (1944–45) to state that there was no discussion "in the literature of the evaluation and interpretation of the pathologic process of demyelinating diseases in the human brain in the light of allergic reactions." Taking the contrast between degenerative and inflammatory theories of the disease as a false one, Ferraro attempted to unify the many suggested etiologies (infectious, toxic, lipolytic, vascular) under the single phenomenon of allergy. He argued that many of the factors said experimentally to induce demyelination actually induce an allergic reaction and that the vascular events known to occur in the lesions can be attributed to an allergic reaction. This position had the advantage of giving the by then enormous diversity of agents a single primary focus. Whether the reaction was anaphylactic (due to a prior sensitization) or generally allergic (due to any destructive interaction between antigens and antibodies), the pathology was the same.

Putnam himself had suggested allergy as an explanation of the thrombotic processes, and the proposed adoption of allergy as a covering concept to an extent vindicated his vascular researches. The creation of Schilder's disease early in the century began an increasingly fine "confusion" of new clinicopathological entities (Ferraro 1944:476) lacking experimental verification or clinical usefulness. Thus Ferraro and his colleagues continued the trend identified by Sachs and Friedman, away from the old late stage study of lesions and toward an examination of lesion development through experimentation. Rejecting even current European efforts to identify infectious agents behind MS, they addressed demyelinating diseases as a whole. They reflected a wish in medicine to find the most general cause and the most broadly effective treatment.

Ferraro, the Kopeloffs and many of their colleagues were of European origin working in the United States and forwarding a research project that had begun as a break with European approaches to MS. Like researchers in the nuclear physics research taking place at the same time in the United States, some of the most prolific researchers were from nations engaged in World War II, raging at the time. As George Hassin wrote in the introduction to the first number of the *Journal of Neuropathology and Experimental Neurology* (1942:2): "Due to the sad conditions in Europe now, largely a veritable vacuum as far as science is concerned, activities in research are bound to be centered in this country." There follows an article on MS pathology by the German émigré Otto Marburg, who had contributed greatly both to the "confusion" of diagnostic types and to the possibility of its resolution through experiment. Ferraro's article freely cites Italian and German research where relevant while explicitly rejecting some of the old conclusions. He also recalls some of the U.S. research that led to his own proclamation of cerebral demyelination as an allergic reaction of the brain. Charcot had begun his clinicopathological summary of *sclérose en plaques*, some 70 years earlier, with a history of the investigations that his work capped. Ferraro attempted to create a history for his own experimental pathology.

Experimental allergic encephalomyelitis or encephalopathy was the chief product of the process-oriented researches given impetus by the 1921 New

York meeting. The relationship between the animal models and human cerebral disease was debated during the following years, leading to many variants of the experimental allergic encephalopathy (EAE) demonstration and many interpretations of the results. EAE did have the effect of establishing an experimental method that could be used to advance neurological arguments and project therapies. At the very least, it provided a way to produce tissue samples under controlled conditions, which could then be compared with MS and other cerebral disease tissue using increasingly sophisticated imaging techniques (electron microscopy). Researchers varied EAE to learn how to produce MS lesions in animals, presumably reflecting similar processes in humans.

Surveying several decades of MS research employing EAE, C. E. Lumsden (1958:754) wrote "Whatever the pathogenesis of allergic encephalomyelitis, the fact is that no experimental instance has, to my knowledge, been published or illustrated which reproduces demyelinating lesions in any way approaching the characteristic lesions of multiple sclerosis which I think it is important to re-examine regularly if one is to keep one's sense of perspective." Though EAE had been a valuable tool for the study of immune reactions in tissue, its chemistry was still not specified. And Hassin's objection to Putnam's experimental lesions still was in force: the lesions produced artificially were not the same as MS lesions. Lumsden was calling for a careful comparison of real MS lesions with EAE lesions. But all too often in the ensuing years it was assumed that the lesions produced by the established techniques of EAE were the same as MS lesions. Neglecting the pathology so meticulously laid out by Charcot, Dawson, Hassin, Marburg and others led to equating "experimental MS lesions" with EAE lesions not strongly resembling MS.

Some researchers, like A. Wolf, E. A. Kabat and A. E. Bezer (1946) were careful to make only general comparisons between EAE and human demyelinating disease, a category in which MS was included. But the assumption of the similarity between EAE and MS slipped in through matching of myelin damage patterns (Wisniewski 1972) in both conditions. A dogma of MS as demyelinating disease was in part sustained by the uncritical pursuit of EAE trials. Replacing "allergic" with "autoimmune" in EAE gave the model deep connections to other developments in biochemistry and neurology.

The validity of EAE as a model for MS turned on accepting MS as a demyelinating disease and ignoring other factors. It was a valuable model for directing research into primary causes and treatment of the lesion itself. But even as myelin was analyzed chemically and its formation replicated in the laboratory, objections arose to the primacy of demyelination in MS and thus to the etiologies and treatments based on lesions. P. B. James (1982 quoted by Betts 1988:4) faulted contemporary accounts of MS for leaving out a host of other conditions that don't fit into the myelin-loss model: loss of neurons, involvement of peripheral nerves, petechiae (sudden bursts or spots) in the skin and other vascular changes. There was no study of the source of the lesions themselves or their distribution. EAE gave the lesions artificially induced in animals an MS character and led to the ignoring of the attributes of the disease in humans.

Frederick Wolfgram (1979:3) gave a terse summary of EAE's effect on MS research. "Three decades of myopic preoccupation with EAE have resulted in limiting our investigations almost exclusively to immunology and virology, although either discipline has yet to offer a credible explanation of the etiology of MS." EAE long remained the defining procedure for the study of MS and the technique that was taught to physicians and researchers in training for how to visualize the action of the disease. This even carried over into new envisionments, such as evoked potential and MRI. But other histories of MS were beginning.

12

The Swayback Workers

Sometimes a newborn lamb or young sheep loses its bounding spring, staggers about with back curved down and succumbs to paralysis, or it never rises at all from its birthing fall. Shepherds and farmers in England had recognized this affliction for some time and gave it the name "warfa" or "swayback." It occurred more frequently and with greater intensity in some areas, such as Derbyshire, Yorkshire, Buckinghamshire and Wales; and it fluctuated from year to year, in some years afflicting nearly all of the lambs. Sheep-producing Australia and New Zealand also saw swayback, as did Peru, Argentina and South Africa, but it was not reported from America or from Europe, apart possibly from Sweden.

Researchers from the Cambridge University Institute of Animal Pathology, urged to find a way to prevent this problem from curbing domestic sheep production, began studying the disease in the mid 1920s. They learned that there were distinct affected areas in Great Britain in which swayback mortality was much higher than in contiguous areas. Ewes who had spent at least a year in one of these areas, though healthy at the time, were more likely to bear swayback lambs than other ewes. Single lambs, twins and triplets all could have the disease.

Beginning work in 1934, J. R. M. Innes, a veterinarian, determined that swayback had a demyelinating pathology accompanied by degeneration of the motor tracts. The nerve tissue became softened, in some cases to the point of liquefaction of a portion of the cerebral hemisphere. Innes compared the swayback pathology with Schilder's encephalopathy in humans (Campbell et al. 1947:50). By that time there was reason to do so.

Many attempts to transfer swayback from infected animals to the unexposed or to laboratory animals ended in failure. Eventually researchers learned that swayback could be prevented by giving the animals copper supplements. The precise cause of the disease remained elusive.

145

In December 1938 one of the veterinary scientists who worked on the 1936 experiment saw Dr. W. Ritchie Russell, a neurologist at Oxford's Radcliffe Infirmary. He told the doctor that the previous June he had experienced difficulty walking and could not chase the ball while playing tennis. This had ceased to trouble him after a few days; what brought him to the neurologist was a relapse two weeks earlier. His legs, especially the right one, were again slowed and had the same sensation as in June. The third, fourth and fifth fingers of his right hand also were numbed. Only the fingers were found to have abnormal discrimination of sensation (two points of touch) during the neurological examination. And the triceps reflexes were much less active. Other than that, all the sensations and muscle reflexes were normal. He had a negative Wassermann test, and syphilis could be dismissed as a cause. The man's sister had died of disseminated sclerosis at age 35. Dr. Russell thought this might be the early stages of the same disease. An occurrence of retrobulbar neuritis in 1939, which cleared up six weeks later, tended to confirm the diagnosis.

Another of the workers on the same team had some sensory symptoms as early as mid–1938, and by 1939 his legs were weakened. He began to suffer periodic attacks of weakness in one or more of his limbs, which then partially recovered. This became a permanent spastic paresis in all four limbs; together with vision loss, this led two London neurologists to give a diagnosis of disseminated sclerosis.

In a paper on experimental production of demyelination in animals, Innes and Shearer (1940) listed the many agents that could be made to induce demyelination in animals. These demonstrations simply showed that demyelination has a variety of potential causes, not that any one cause is primary. They mentioned the encephalitis known to occur in the aftermath of infectious disease in humans and animals but did not see this as an adequate explanation of human demyelination. They mentioned that several of the men who had taken part in the 1936–38 swayback study were suffering from conditions of the central nervous system.

Having had success discovering a measure to prevent a serious demyelinating condition in animals, Innes, at the end of World War II, put together a team to study "disseminated sclerosis ... the only common demyelinating disease of humans" (Campbell et al. 1947:53). Incorporating physicians, geologists and chemists, this was to be a local and international study that would pin down environmental factors, as the swayback study had done before the war. "A new line of approach opened up when it was found that the number of swayback research workers suffering from a disease of the central nervous system had reached remarkable proportions."

No fewer than four of the seven principal workers in a swayback research unit had come down with these conditions. The authors of the report gave brief case descriptions of the three workers showing symptoms by 1940, all of them still with some symptoms associated with disseminated sclerosis. The fourth one was added in 1946 when he saw Dr. Russell; he had an intermittent dragging of his left leg and some exaggerated or diminished reflexes exposed by neurological examination. The authors of the article were careful to refer to the "disease of the central nervous system" of the four workers, but in their discussion they found clear evidence of "multiple lesions with the remissions and relapses which the neurologist stresses so strongly in the diagnosis of disseminated sclerosis."

This cluster of cases was sufficient to lead them to tabulate qualities the four men had in common: they were roughly the same age, and the first three affected, in 1938–39, were of Scottish birth and upbringing. Two were research biochemists doing analyses of blood, tissues, soil and pastures, one (Case 2) succeeding the other (Case 1) at this work and both having extensive contact with swayback materials and one (Case 2) of them also handling live affected sheep as late as 1946. Another (Case 3) was an agricultural advisory officer involved in the swayback field studies and had handled a number of live cases in 1937–39. The latest man affected (Case 4) was a laboratory technician assisting the two biochemists over several decades.

Innes himself was one of the three unaffected workers, despite handling many hundreds of living swayback cases and performing over 250 autopsies. Some exposed to swayback contracted disseminated sclerosis. Extent or kind of exposure (blood or live animals) didn't seem to make any difference.

Apart from the demyelination and resulting incoordination, disseminated sclerosis in humans and swayback in lambs are more dissimilar than alike. They do not seem to be human and animal versions of the same disease. Both diseases have peculiar patterns of geographical distribution, but there is nothing in that to connect them with each other. The researchers looked for what the four affected workers might have shared in the workplace, for example possibly exposure to a toxic factor in the laboratory. But not all of those affected worked in the laboratory. Possibly a copper deficiency in humans led to a viral infection that caused demyelinating disease or vice versa. Or it may have been a deficiency of other trace elements separately or in combination. Four out of seven men involved in studies of swayback came down with disseminated sclerosis. There was nothing to explain why these four men were ill and why others on the same projects, with the same exposures and of similar age and origins, did not suffer.

The biochemist who showed the clearest signs of MS (designated Case 1 by A. M. G. Campbell) died in 1953 at the age of 49. After his initial walking impairment, he was suffering from a variety of movement (pyramidal and cerebellar) and visual symptoms by 1947 and was bedridden by 1950. He died of bronchial pneumonia secondary to the neurological disease. C. E. Lumsden, a pathologist at the University of Leeds, performed the autopsy (1958:752). The man's MS "by a curious coincidence only — happened to be of a rather transitional type with diffuse cerebral demyelination and with plaques of the more typical discrete type only in the optic pathway, cerebellum, brain stem and cord."

The "curious coincidence" was between the pathology of Case 1's MS and the diffuse demyelination characteristic of swayback. Lumsden did not believe that the case had anything at all to do with "the swayback problem." He began his article referring to the prominence that the four cases of MS among swayback workers had received in the world literature on demyelinating disease. At that time, ten years after Campbell et al. made their report, the time had come for a reassessment. The one case that had come to autopsy did show signs of this peculiar MS, but Lumsden was implicitly skeptical about any relationship between MS and infectious disease that could be deduced from it. "If we were to learn that the diagnosis of multiple sclerosis is no longer tenable in the remaining cases cited in the 1947 report I think it would be of real value in the difficult field of multiple sclerosis research." That finally would disentangle MS from swayback.

In Lumsden's article there seems almost an impatience about the swayback workers. If there was no clustering of MS among them, then a strong and frequently cited piece of evidence for communicable MS would be disqualified. For a pathologist, there was no way to be sure until after their deaths.

In 1954 Case 3, the advisory officer, died at the age of 45 after having been blind in one eye and without the use of his legs for about a year. He had first come to Campbell in 1939 with a localized lesion of the spinal cord that manifested as weakness in the right leg and thermal disturbances. The examining physician diagnosed focal myelitis. The patient asked if the condition might have been caused by a blow from a tennis ball on the spine. He recovered from this, but two or three minor relapses seem to have followed minor accidents. In 1945 he went to an ophthalmologist with a complaint of hazy vision. The discovery of a scotoma led the man himself to believe that he had retrobulbar neuritis and that it must be an early sign of disseminated sclerosis. When a neurologist examined him later in 1945 there was no loss of coordination, and though the plantar reflexes were extensor (normal), he did not have an abdominal reflex. The right eye was shaky when he looked to the right, and an ophthalmoscopic examination showed a pallor on the temporal half of the right optic disc. The specialist found it "very probable" that he was in "the very early stages of disseminated sclerosis." Both the weakness in his legs and the loss of vision in his right eye continued for the remaining eight years of his life and intensified a year before his death. The listed cause of death was a perforated duodenal ulcer. No necropsy was performed.

The biochemist (Case 2) who had succeeded Case 1 in his job died in 1955 at age 52 of hemorrhaging after stomach surgery to correct a chronic duodenal ulcer. He had not seen his own doctor about neurological symptoms between his first sensory symptoms of 1938 and his death, but after his death his wife wrote to Campbell (1963:514) telling him that her husband had experienced mild neurological symptoms and was convinced that he had disseminated sclerosis. There was no necropsy in his case either.

The lead author of the 1947 paper that first brought the swayback workers to medical attention wrote a follow-up of the cases (Campbell 1963) after the three had died. The one surviving man (Case 4) had begun to show symptoms (difficulty walking, spasticity of both legs) of MS only in 1946. Since then, he had become incapacitated with spasticity and movement (cerebellar) disturbances and had lost the sight of one eye entirely and partially that of the other. When Campbell examined the man in 1961, he found "gross cerebellar defect, gross spasticity and bilaterial optic atrophy."

The cerebrospinal fluid test showed a "paretic Lange curve," which confirmed the diagnosis of disseminated sclerosis. This test result was a change from the same man's 1946 negative Lange test. The gold test was originally devised by the Danish chemist Karl Georg Lange (1834–1900) to evaluate central nervous system damage due to syphilis, and since D. K. Smith's work in the early 1920s, it had been used in Great Britain as an assay for disseminated sclerosis. Campbell had not adopted Elvin Kabat's definitive 1947 MS test based on oligoclonal bands in cerebrospinal fluid, but he relied on the assumption that MS has syphilitic underpinnings to confirm the disease with a positive Lange reading.

Campbell was acutely aware of the lack of pathological data to support the common diagnosis of disseminated sclerosis in two of the three deceased swayback workers. He made arrangements to have a necropsy performed "if possible" when the remaining man died. But any argument that all four had disseminated sclerosis would forever be based on clinical symptoms and personal guesswork. Swayback itself was known to be a deficiency disease in sheep and not infective; that all four came down with their disease of the central nerve system after working on swayback seemed to be coincidental. It may have been a human disease that spread among them because they were associated with each other. One of the workers — Case 2 in the 1947 article — had a sister who had died of disseminated sclerosis: possibly he had infected the others with the causative agent. To Campbell, the four cases strengthened the possibility that disseminated sclerosis is due to an unknown virus, but in the summary of his article he concluded that "no reasonable explanation" for the cluster of cases had yet been found.

Lumsden was not certain that all four workers had disseminated sclerosis. By the time of Campbell's 1963 paper, it had become impossible to determine that for sure. After reviewing this (lack of) evidence, Campbell still treated the four cases as an unexplained cluster of disseminated sclerosis. This cluster offered a epidemiological phrasing of the MS problem too tempting to overlook. Though Campbell didn't mention it in his 1965 paper, Case 4, the only one still alive at that time, was thoroughly examined at the National

Hospital, London, by a number of neurologists, most of whom concluded that
he had disseminated sclerosis. Dr. Macdonald Critchley gave the opinion that
the man was suffering from "human swayback." One of those favoring disseminated sclerosis was Charles P. Symonds, who referred to the cases in his
article "Multiple Sclerosis and the Swayback Story" (1975). By that time, Case
4 had died (in December 1966) and a full necropsy had been done, but
Symonds did not seem to be aware of it. He asked if the diagnosis of MS had
been confirmed by pathological examination of any of the cases reported in
1947. A detailed pathology of Case 4's tissue and of prepared slides of brain
material did show changes considered characteristic of MS (Dean, McDougall
and Elian 1985:862). But Symonds did not know about the earlier cases that
Campbell had reported in his 1965 article.

Unlike Lumsden, who performed a necropsy on some of the tissue of
Case 1, or Campbell, who had tried to watch development over 20 years,
Symonds was interested in applying an emergent theory of MS pathogenesis
to the swayback workers. He referred to recent studies suggesting that a slow
virus precipitated an autoimmune reaction to yield the "clinical and pathological features of multiple sclerosis." He thus combined two new medical
hypotheses to explain the relationship between the demyelinating disease of
sheep and that of humans.

Slow viruses, manifesting over very long periods, had been postulated by
Carleton Gajdusek as the cause of a number of degenerative diseases of the
brain, including kuru of a New Guinea people, Creutzfeld-Jakob disease of
Europeans, scrapie of sheep and spongiform encephalopathy of cows. The
autoimmune concept had been put forward to account for cellular damage that
could not be explained as the direct result of infection. Some initiating cause
would make the immune system read body tissues as invaders to be destroyed.
A virus, especially a slow virus, could precipitate this reaction, which would
then continue unchecked. This pairing of virus and autoimmune reaction married endogenous and exogenous causes of MS, causes that had been debated
over the previous decades. It was a way of expanding the previously popular
theory of MS as allergy, a reaction to a foreign substance, by making an outside, communicable factor the cause of an internal allergic response. It was a
way of including both the internally degenerative and the infectious qualities
of MS pathology and epidemiology.

With this explanation as the prize, Symonds was motivated to seek a slow
virus in swayback. He questioned the conclusion that swayback is a copper
deficiency only, but he returned to the suggestion of Campbell and colleagues
that it might be caused by an infective agent in the presence of a copper
deficiency. But there were no studies to support the speculation. He discounted
a slow virus alone as the cause of the MS among the swayback workers. For
the first time in any of the swayback-MS papers, he mentioned that there had
not been MS outbreaks in other groups of swayback workers. If a slow virus

was to be preserved as the possible infectious factor, then another event peculiar to this group had to be postulated. Symonds postulated that the slow virus is very widespread in the population and produces asymptomatic myelin degeneration. Encountering the myelin degeneration products in the sheep materials they were handling may have incited an autoimmune reaction to the workers' own myelin affected by the virus. The MS-affected sister of one of the men might indicate a genetic factor disposed to this immunological reaction.

Symonds's conception of an autoimmune reaction is actually autoallergic, derived from earlier ideas of MS as an allergic reaction to alien or self-factors. His slow virus–autoimmune theory, as he recognized, is too general to explain the clustering of disease among the swayback four. He postulated further that there is still an undetected additional component in their disease. Environmental conditions or practices for handling research materials handling practices may show the decisive difference. The fate of the swayback workers is still an open question attracting the latest theories as they develop.

Geoffrey Dean, E. I. McDougall and M. Elian (1985) begin their discussion of the swayback cases stating what continues to be true: "It is difficult to find a common cause that could apply to all four cases of multiple sclerosis as well as applying to those who did not develop the disease." Using the same numbering as Campbell, Dean and colleagues reviewed each of the four cases and adduced information supplementary to and, to some extent, contradicting what Campbell, Lumsden and Symonds had offered. Worker 1 (Patient 1 or Case 1) is now shown in the full severity of the symptoms he suffered after his relapse in 1940. By the time he was admitted to Radcliffe Infirmary, Oxford, under Dr. Russell's care in 1947, he was "disorientated, mentally confused and incapable of sustained conversation."

> He was temperamentally aggressive but there was euphoria. He had slurring of speech, incoordination of his arms and legs, diminution of vibration sense in his legs, spasticity in all of his limbs, the plantar responses were extensor, his knee and ankle tendon reflexes were brisk and the abdominal reflexes were absent. He had a pleural effusion following a previous haemothorax resulting from a fall. He gave his age as 32 when he was, in fact, 42. Efforts to help him walk with a walking aid were not successful.

The Wasserman test was negative, and the Lange gold curve was normal: no syphilis was involved. Campbell's 1947 report, based on the same neurological records, was much more circumspect, perhaps to avoid exposure of the man's identity or association with symptoms embarrassing to family members then alive. Admitted to Morningfield Hospital in Aberdeen in July 1951, the man was the same as he had been in 1947 and was "generally unable to do things." A necropsy performed when the man died in 1953 showed an increase of subarachnoid fluid of gelatinous character over both brain hemispheres and an atrophy of the gyri. The brain, spinal cord and other materials were removed and sent to Lumsden for further examination. Though he promised a more detailed account of the pathology of this worker when he mentioned the case in the 1965 article, Lumsden did not publish anything further. An intensive search of both hospital and home records did not yield Lumsden's notes on these specimens, but he did write Campbell a letter saying that he would not say much more about it but that he had found "extensive foci of demyelination." To the professor of pathology at Aberdeen, Lumsden also remarked that his findings were "very similar to that of Schilder's disease."

Worker 2 had a much less severe case of weakness in his limbs, developing around the same time as Worker 1 suffered his symptoms. Dean's revision is not much more detailed than Campbell's original account because there was not much more to reveal from records and there was no necropsy. Worker 2's sister was said to have died of disseminated sclerosis and was even proposed as a possible source of an infection, but family members recalled to Dean that she had died of tuberculosis. The course of Worker 2's illness makes the diagnosis of disseminated sclerosis "acceptable," but there was no family history of the disease.

Dean and his colleagues also interviewed relatives of Worker 3 and picked up confirmation that he had walked with a swaying gait. This, in addition to the physicians' record of extensor plantar response, lack of abdominal reflexes and loss of vision, substantiated the disseminated sclerosis diagnosis. From his widow they learned that he had fallen from the platform of a bus in 1947 and injured his head. After that, his walking slowly deteriorated, leading to his retirement in 1953 and an even more rapid failure of both walking and mental functions. There was no necropsy, but "probable multiple sclerosis would appear to have been the correct diagnosis."

The most thorough account was of Worker 4, whose necropsy had been carefully arranged before his death in 1966 at the age of 60. He had reflex weakness and "slight but definite intellectual impairment" when tested in 1950. His positive Wasserman test and an "abnormal" Lange gold curve at that time both implied syphilis, discreetly left unnamed. Postmortem, his brain contained scattered pink plaques and a generalized reduction of the white matter. Gelatinous grey areas in the medulla and a number of grey patches scattered along the spinal cord, added to the plaques, gliosis and loss of myelin visible under the microscope, completed the picture gained by studies immediately after his death. In 1981, fifteen years later, Professor Ingrid Allen, a histopathologist at Queen's University, Belfast, examined slides of brain and spine materials and found areas of demyelination, intense glial reaction and various other tissue changes that indicated inflammatory demyelinating disease with a histology quite compatible with some forms of multiple sclerosis.

The clinical history and necropsies led to an "undoubted diagnosis" of multiple sclerosis.

Soon after Worker 4 died, part of his brain was sent to an experimental pathology laboratory in Iceland, where a preparation made from it was injected into the brains of five sheep "to see if it would induce scrapie" (not swayback). It didn't, and when the last of the sheep was slaughtered in 1979 there was no sign or evidence of scrapie in the brain.

On the other hand a survey of humans who had worked on swayback in England, Scotland, Australia, New Zealand and South Africa, a total of 50 in all, did not turn up a single case of MS during the years between 1938 and 1984. There was one case of motor neurone disease (ALS).

This was a final, thorough examination of all the remaining records of the four Cambridge-Derbyshire workers in swayback who came down with MS. The researchers once again dismissed the possibility that the MS might have been "human swayback" despite the swayback-like pathology of only one worker (Case 1). Dean and colleagues added one worker who joined the swayback research late but never came down with MS. Using the higher prevalence rate of the disease calculated for the part of Scotland from which two of the men came, they determined the likelihood that four men out of eight would come down with MS to be about one in one thousand million. This suggested that some other factor was at work tilting the odds in favor of infection. Because the four worked together in the same place on the sheep disease and had the same kind of infection, it seems most likely that an environmental and or infectious factor was at work.

Dean and colleagues mentioned, as Campbell had, that there was a possibility that all four had been exposed to lead, a well-known slow neural poison. But there was no evidence of that beyond the circumstantial. No one had tested the pathology samples for excess lead. They did not even refer to the repeated suggestion that transmission of pathogens be studied in an environment of copper deficiency: that seems to have been forgotten entirely.

Symonds's slow virus–autoimmune theory did not come up at all. Instead Dean and colleagues attributed to Symonds a causative factor that he didn't actually introduce: encephalitogenic (brain-breaking) protein. Perhaps they were confusing Symonds with Lumsden, who was the coauthor of a study of the protein in the spinal cord (Carnegie and Lumsden 1966). The protein was of interest because it had been implicated in scrapie, another disease of sheep, and scrapie in turn had been associated symptomatically and pathologically with MS by a group of researchers that included the neurologist Campbell of the 1947 swayback paper (Dick, McAlister, McKeown and Campbell 1965).

Encephalitogenic protein was found in the mid–1960s to be a peptide that could behave as if it were a virus under some circumstances, producing encephalitis symptoms and neuropathology and passing infectiously from one host to another. It was the "slow virus" that Gajdusek had found behind kuru and Creutzfeld-Jakob disease in humans. By the time of Dean et al.'s 1985 article, Tikvah Alper and her team at Hammersmith Hospital in London had found that the scrapie agent lacks nucleic acids and could be degraded by ultraviolet light. The brain samples were sent to Iceland for P. A. Palsson, a specialist in slow viruses, to determine if the MS of the swayback workers was caused by the same agent that caused scrapie. That turned out to be a dead end, and while research into the molecular biology of scrapie matured in the late 1980s, there were no swayback worker brain samples available for further study and testing. The suspicion of "slow viruses" in MS was sufficient for those studying an "epidemic" of MS on the Orkney and Shetland Islands to try to correlate cases with consumption of an animal brain dish, "potted head" (Poskanzer et al. 1980). The role of "infectious amyloid" or of "prions" in MS remains to be seen (Wojtowicz 1993).

Between their first appearance in the literature in 1940 and the most recent in 1985, the swayback cases went through an evolution apart from the development of their personal affliction. The belief that they had a common ailment went from a "disease of the central nervous system" to "demyelinating disease" to "disseminated sclerosis" or "multiple sclerosis" even as the diversity of their symptoms became clear and even after one autopsy showed a pathology only marginally consistent with the judgment of MS.

After the autopsy of the fourth case, Dean and his coauthors still referred to them as four cases of MS even though the fourth worker had tested positive on the standard tests for syphilis. If he were an isolated case, his symptoms probably would have been interpreted as neurosyphilis. The first worker to die and the only one of the first three to have an autopsy died of Schilder's disease, with a pathology of cerebral softening that the turn-of-the-century pathologists classified in contradistinction to the patchy hardening of MS. The resemblance of his tissue to swayback tissue seems to have fixed him as an MS victim who was exposed to swayback, and no amount of new information changed this.

The other two workers had "probable" cases of MS based on a few symptoms, and they themselves seem to have been convinced that they were suffering from the disease. MS diagnostics was being standardized from the beginning of the century, but the physicians who viewed and reviewed these cases, as well as the men themselves during their lifetimes, seem to have been charmed by the thought of a clue to MS. They could dismiss a direct link to swayback but not the very broad covering category of MS. Case 2's sister died of TB, it turned out, but the possibility of cerebrospinal TB never was considered.

Though there was a call for autopsies, they were not done. The ability of Charcot to hold his patients from diagnosis to autopsy for the sake of the clinicopathological method was not reproduced in pre–national health plan Great Britain. The one researcher with the greatest overview of the cases,

A. M. G. Campbell, does not seem to have followed them, though he was very interested in the effects of animal diseases on humans. And Lumsden, perhaps the most critical intelligence among those involved with the cases, either never produced or mislaid his analysis of the cellular pathology of the one worker who died during his lifetime.

The swayback workers continue to be mentioned in the MS literature as a singular clustering of MS in an occupational group and as a hint that MS might somehow be primarily infectious in nature. The role of environment in MS is also mentioned. Yet no one has attempted to correlate this set of cases with others in the same area around the same time or with others from the same areas of origin. MS does not cluster among swayback workers as such, but does it cluster in other occupational groups in Derbyshire?

A number of treatments for MS were proposed and tested during the 30 years of the swayback workers' illness, but there is no record of any of these treatments being administered. Even symptomatic treatment goes unmentioned in the accounts of the cases. Some of the authors were treating neurologists, and it is hard to believe that those afflicted did not seek relief. But even that aspect of their humanity is absent from the accounts. They remain epidemiological models and an etiological conundrum, the ideal suffering bodies of an idealized disease.

13

MS Goes Public

On October 25, 1942, the *New York Times* reported Tracy Putnam's statement at the American Medical Association meeting that MS is due to faulty blood clotting. At that time, Putnam was considering a newly discovered drug, dicoumarin, as a treatment. Dicoumarin had been isolated from spoiled sweet clover in 1941 and found to be of use in reducing blood clots. Firmly convinced by his experiments that MS was a result of thrombosis of blood vessels feeding nerve tissue, Putnam sought an effective anticoagulant to free up the blood flow. He did not believe that histamine, a subject of experimental treatments at the Mayo Clinic and elsewhere, was lasting in its effects.

Putnam's actual use of dicoumarin for his own patients and his suggestions to referring physicians became cautious as he completed clinical trials of the drug (Putnam, Chiavacci, Hoff and Weitzen 1947) and moved to the West Coast, establishing a large specialty practice in Los Angeles. Dicoumarin was mainly of use in acute relapses to reduce the "prothrombin time" (blood-clotting time) of a patient (Talley 1995:47).

Putnam's experimental work and his advice on drugs and treatment had long been available to his colleagues and their patients, but his 1942 announcement in the newspaper was the first time the *New York Times* had ever referred to MS in a major article. It was probably the first time many readers had heard about the disease and the research going on into its causes and treatments.

The history of MS up to 1942 had been reported in medical journals, research laboratories, letters and journals. That was the darkest time of World War II for the United States, with the Japanese in control of the western Pacific, the Axis powers dominating continental Europe, and Britain under siege. In Nazi Germany, MS sufferers were grouped in hostels with other invalids and people traumatized by war, where they might be assisted in committing suicide. Putnam's words of encouragement to sufferers of a mysterious disease and the prospect of a drug that had been discovered in and could be manufactured in the United States transcended the obscurity of MS.

After Putnam's announcement, the *New York Times* did not print any articles about MS during the years 1943–46. In 1945, in what now seems like rapid succession, victory was declared in Europe, FDR died, atom bombs were dropped on Hiroshima and Nagasaki and Japan surrendered. On August 12, 1945, there appeared a small classified ad: "Multiple sclerosis. Will anyone recovered from it please communicate with patient?" and there followed the address of Sylvia Lawry. Mrs. Lawry's brother Bernard Friedman had been diagnosed with MS, and their family had not found any viable treatments despite Putnam's announcement. None of the many replies to the ad were from someone who had recovered from MS, but many told of their own or relatives' suffering with the disease, sympathized with the difficulty and asked how they might help bring about a change.

An article in *Newsweek* (1952:47) mentioned the "therapeutic nihilism" of some physicians who told MS patients they had an incurable, untreatable disease. Patients and their families reacted to this hopelessness with a determination that Sylvia Lawry shared and was able to organize. Her work as a court reporter and consumer advocate over the radio gave her experience in the preparation of briefs and the use of broadcast media. She was able to channel the energies of the war effort into a war against disease.

A president who himself suffered from polio, Franklin D. Roosevelt, had lent his support to the creation (1938) of a national charity, the National Foundation for Infantile Paralysis (March of Dimes), to collect funds for research into treatment of polio, and he had sponsored legislation to form a government program charged with reducing polio casualties. There already was a national cancer research institute within the National Institutes of Health. When Sylvia Lawry and her sister Ruth Friedman convened meetings of those who had responded to the 1945 advertisement, they had in the polio and cancer institutions an excellent model for planning collective action.

On February 22, 1946, the *Times* published an article on the incidence of MS; on August 11, Putnam gave the not entirely encouraging results of his group study of dicoumarin for MS; and on October 3, Sylvia Lawry and her sister announced the formation of the Association for the Advancement of Research on Multiple Sclerosis.

The following year the association changed its name to the more manageable National Multiple Sclerosis Society (NMSS), appointed a medical director and awarded its first three research grants. Now having a distinct organization to serve as a source of information, the *Times* began to print news of MS research, the opening of MS clinics and MS society activities. Other local newspapers in cities with clinics strongly involved in MS research — Boston and St. Louis, Missouri — had mentioned MS occasionally before this, but the national society provided a national focus for news about MS.

A popular science periodical with a national circulation, *Science News Letter*, made its first mention of the disease on October 26, 1947, when it reported the formation of the society.

There was no public celebrity with MS to serve as a rallying point and certification of the movement as FDR did for polio research. But a celebrity would not have been enough. When baseball star Lou Gehrig retired from the game (1939), having been paralyzed by amyptrophic lateral sclerosis (ALS), Americans began to call the disease by his name and, after his death in 1941, contributed to a national research fund headed by his widow. Yet this was not enough to create a drive against ALS. The number of people afflicted with MS, the much greater number of friends and family members obliged to watch helplessly the growing disability and the lack of any effective treatment even as penicillin seemed to wipe out syphilis, created a community of well-situated backers for public action against MS.

Senator Charles W. Tobey of New Hampshire sponsored the National Multiple Sclerosis Act, which began hearings before the Senate Subcommittee on Health of the Committee on Labor and Public Welfare on May 10, 1949. Senator Tobey's own daughter had multiple sclerosis, and he sought the advice of the National Multiple Sclerosis Society in composing the legislation. When the proposal for a National Multiple Sclerosis Research Institute was included in hearings on a National Health Plan in the House of Representatives in 1949, Ralph I. Straus, the president of the National Multiple Sclerosis Society, gave testimony, as did Senator Tobey, Mrs. Lou Gehrig and Dr. Tracy Putnam, as well as a number of other doctors, family members and patients.

They were not entirely in agreement. Most of the laypeople present stated that no progress whatsoever had been made in the "fight" against MS and demanded the kind of government intervention that had made possible the mass production of penicillin, which in turn was credited for the sustained health of Allied troops invading Nazi Europe. Putnam, who had been an active participant in MS research for the last two decades, was confronted by a discontented public who did not seem to know about the progress he and others had achieved since Cruveilhier and Carswell.

Putnam was the first major researcher to go public with a theory of MS causes and the prospect of a treatment in 1942, but in 1949 he could not claim great success for this treatment. Though he described further research into other medications, he was facing people who wanted results, not hypotheses. He also was in private practice and had seen the devastation of lives and the suicide brought on by the diagnosis of MS (e.g., the young California man with MS who shot himself in the chest after going blind in one eye; Talley 1995:52 n. 138 from Putnam's exam records).

In 1948 the Columbia University researcher Elvin Kabat, one of the first recipients of a NMSS grant, announced the discovery of antibodies in cerebrospinal fluid indicative of pathological processes associated with MS and other demyelinating diseases. Kabat had already published several joint papers of experimental allergic encephalopathy studies, but his proposal to the NMSS focused on seeking a diagnostic test. The oligoclonal bands that he and his team found were more characteristic of MS pathology than the Lange gold test and were one more dissociation of MS from syphilis.

The NMSS came to the Senate and House hearings with evidence that its approach to MS research could foster constructive diagnostic and treatment tools where the medical profession, left to its own devices, had failed. Consumer funding and consumer criteria were beginning to dictate the priorities of medical research. Charcot's ability simply to study the disease of those accepted as doomed could no longer be the ideal of medical research. Projecting that ideal into animals was only a stopgap measure. The patients and their representatives were demanding control of the expenditure of private and public money for research on MS.

The realities of federal bureaucracy made it impossible to establish a national institute for a single neurological disease. The advocates had to settle for studies undertaken by the National Institute of Mental Health and some partial government subsidy of university research. The national society itself had become a major fund-raiser for research. Through a medical director and grant-application review panels, the society was able to influence the direction of research.

Research was a component in the larger work of the society: to make available information about MS to health professionals, patients and the wider public. The need for information stemmed from the organizers' understanding of the consequences of MS being an obscure yet, as they saw it, ever more frequently diagnosed disease. "Medical compassion" or just ignorance often caused doctors to keep those diagnosed in the dark about the findings, perhaps telling only the family. This had been the practice from earlier in the century (recall Barbellion), and it only contributed to the dark repute of the disease. The University of Chicago education professor John Robert Ginther published a personal account of MS (1978); he described the effects of not being told about his own MS (diagnosed 1962) for ten years while his family knew about it.

This hesitancy to name the disease also made it difficult for patients to communicate with each other and support each other in the face of a highly uncertain personal future. There was no basis for collective action against employers who fired those with MS and no way to demand special consideration from public services. Once it had public attention and a research fund, the NMSS attempted to remove the stigma from MS resulting from its obscurity.

One of the society's first publications was a diagnostic manual written by a committee of doctors under the chairmanship of Tracy Putnam and distributed only to doctors. This was the beginning of the society's attempts to define and regularize diagnosis. Respecting the confidentiality of diagnosis was the only way to gain physicians' allegiance to the aims of the society. But in its early education work, the society also countered the isolation that a diagnosis of MS was known to create; it published pamphlets for newly diagnosed patients and their families, synthesizing for the first time MS epidemiology and patient history information that could only prove reassuring to those who had just their doctor's word and rumor to rely on.

Administrators at the March of Dimes, where Sylvia Lawry first sought funding and advice, had warned her not to rely on the doctors to raise money. Donations at first came from wealthy philanthropists and were acknowledged in public statements. Like the March of Dimes, the NMSS was primarily funded by large numbers of small donations from people who were described as members of the organization. These members were an audience for the society's guardedly optimistic view of MS. They also could serve to distribute society information, and as the society became national they formed local branches. The second branch formed after New York was in Los Angeles, the Southern California Multiple Sclerosis Society. Though this area was not then the second most heavily populated after New York — it took much longer for an MS society to form in Chicago — it was an object of strong national migration. Both physicians and refugees from harsher climates to the north, people already or likely to become MS patients, moved into the Los Angeles area after the war. Tracy Putnam, in his Los Angeles practice after 1947, received referrals from all over Southern California and from all over the country. The MS society and practices like his in Southern California formed an early center for the dissemination of MS information throughout the western region.

This information took the form of pamphlets on MS for patients and relatives; these were distributed through the mails and by physicians. It was obvious, however, that using this method, the NMSS would reach only those who already had contact with the society or with a physician. To dramatize publicly the need for action against MS and to mobilize new members, the national society began an information campaign through widely distributed periodicals.

Sylvia Lawry's family and professional contacts with executives in New York's burgeoning postwar advertising industry helped place articles in both general-distribution news magazines and more specialized health and science journals. The nature of MS and its victims was conveyed to a wide readership by attaching to the disease a set of words or phrases that called up strong associations. In themselves, the words *multiple sclerosis* were another baffling medical expression for the great majority of readers. The writers and advertisers turned this to their advantage by labeling MS "mysterious," qualifying its unfamiliarity with intrigue and the need to find a solution. If they did not understand scientists' and doctors' approach to MS, the taxpaying public might at least grasp that the disease presented a challenge to these medical detectives.

On October 14, 1946, both *Time* and *Newsweek*, magazines that had not so much as mentioned MS before that date, had brief pieces on the formation of the Association for the Advancement of Research on Multiple Sclerosis, entitled respectively, "Mystery Crippler" and "Mystery of Sclerosis." The disease was "Still a Mystery" for *Time* five years later (December 24, 1951). On November 24, 1952, *Newsweek* printed an article, "Mysterious MS," marking the first use of the initials in a periodical article. Robert J. Grant, with the help of M. Weisinger, declared, "I've Got the Most Mysterious Disease" in the *Saturday Evening Post*, May 22, 1954. Over the years the mystery continued, becoming a specific mystery by 1977 when *Time* (September 5) identified the "MS Mystery: Relationship Between Multiple Sclerosis and Pet Dogs." *New York* magazine reported the "Mystery of MS: Who Gets It and Who Doesn't" on March 26, 1979. It was "MS — Mystery Disease That Strikes the Young" in *U.S. News and World Report* on July 28, 1980, and "Multiple Sclerosis — The Mystery Disease That Baffles Doctors" in *Glamour* for October 1980. "MS — Two New Clues" was in *Science Digest* in August 1979, and on July 28, 1980, *Newsweek* had a "New Clue to the Mystery of MS." On October 6, 1969, *Newsweek* had referred to the "Riddle of MS." In July 1987 it had become "Multiple Sclerosis: A Riddle Wrapped in a Mystery" for C. Shaw in *USA Today*. *Current Health* of that same year told of "Searching for a Key to the Mystery of Multiple Sclerosis," evoking an unrelated metaphor. Colin Talley seemed to cap off this tradition by titling his 1995 history of MS, following the title of Grant's 1954 article, *A Most Mysterious Disease*. The advertisers had succeeded in attaching to MS that single word, with its mood and intention.

If MS was a mystery that baffled the medical profession, it was a foe to be defeated, a battle to be won by the victims and their families. The MS "mystery" stories detailed scientific progress and or befuddlement; the personal stories appearing in an even greater range of journals told of victories over the effects of the disease. These stories reflected a much older tradition of cure narratives, which in the past often had a religious inspiration but which in the MS narratives, as in other American personal-triumph stories, emphasized the skill and determination of the individual overcoming the adversary. This narrative had long been embedded in U.S. public discourse. The publicity challenge was to connect it with MS.

"I escaped a wheelchair," wrote J. C. Benge (*Today's Health*, October 1950). Benge was afflicted with MS, though clearly the disease itself didn't matter so much as the threat of confinement. FDR himself was photographed in a wheelchair only once and stage-managed his public appearances, in the era before television, to be without movement aids of any sort. The recent controversy over his portrayal in a sculptural monument (barely a wheelchair) underlines this sentiment. Leaving the trappings of mechanical support signaled independence recovered through a continuing act of will.

The writer J. Joseph, in the same magazine earlier that year (*Today's Health*, May 1950), described the "sentence commuted" in the lives of several people who, like Benge, had risen from their confinement. Where a diagnosis of MS had previously been a "life-time sentence of physical incapacity," now it was possible to have the sentence commuted to some level of recovery.

There the rehabilitation of one patient began: she was shown exercising at a weight machine. On the surface, this was a contribution to the personal escape-from-MS story, one adopted from the stories of polio and other chronic diseases. The MS society had nurtured the clinic that gave the diagnosis and offered the exercise regimen. But there are several other themes not so far beneath the surface. Instead of receiving a medical treatment, the woman is offered physical therapy that (under guidance and with equipment) can improve her condition. Lacking a treatment that could actually show people recovering from MS once diagnosed, the MS society chose to emphasize the role of exercise. The struggle of those trying to escape MS, or succeed beyond it, could take the form of sit-ups, weight-lifting, running or walking. Exercise was bright, optimistic and photogenic against the passivity and defeatism of the bedridden and the wheelchair-confined. And, of course, exercise really does help energize those who can perform it: that had to be conveyed dramatically.

Sally Mulligan, the subject of a photo article in *Look* magazine (May 18, 1954), was one of the few women with MS shown in the information campaign. She was taken for a habitual drunkard because she staggered on the street, but she found out she had MS when she went to the clinic at Bellevue Hospital in New York supported by the NMSS. Most of the authors and subjects of early MS inspirational stories were men, and men continued to be the focus until quite recently, though women are much more likely to be afflicted. Also diagnostic is the ethnic play in stories like this. Over 70 years earlier, Dr. E. C. Seguin had reported the demise of the whistling Irish accountant Thomas Grogan. Here Sally Mulligan, with her conspicuously Irish name, is thought to be a drunkard until she is revealed to have MS and wins grace through diagnosis and exercise. She then can be shown walking happily on crutches, working as a hospital receptionist, cooking and praying. Transformation from passive female ethnic sufferer into active assimilated and still female combatant is a concealed process of public MS therapy. The article was entitled "Victory in a Wheelchair" and was authored by Raymond Moley, the editor of *Newsweek* magazine.

There was a war going on against MS in the late 1940s and early 1950s. Sylvia Lawry wrote of "Fighting M.S." in *Today's Health* (January 1955). Alongside Sally Mulligan's "Victory in a Wheelchair" was Robert Grant's article "Little Victories" (*Saturday Evening Post*, May 1954). Grant and the article's author, M. Weisinger, compare Grant's learning to walk and handle objects through physical therapy to victories in war — to U.S. victories over "the Nazis and the Nips" in the recent war. As a soldier, Grant had been confined to a wheelchair and had required assistance eating and performing bodily functions, but he had overcome that enemy. Yet the article contains reminders that the battle continued. Another war had begun since the Germans and Japanese were defeated; Stalin was added to the list, and there were allusions to the Cold War. Grant combined the two popular MS images when he described the mystery of the disease as his "Iron Curtain." Yet he is sure that the same science that created antibiotics, isotope therapy and the atomic bomb will defeat MS as well.

The struggle with and triumph over MS that pervades personal and popular scientific accounts of the disease are chilled by a kind of Cold War going on underneath the bright publicity, much as the Cold War itself froze jubilation over victory in World War II. For as many people who escape wheelchairs and have their sentences commuted, there are others with a more qualified optimism. "Today Is What Counts" says J. Sterling in the general magazine *Coronet* (December 1950), telling of his attitude toward his progressive crippling. Janet McCarthy might announce "My Victory Over MS" in *Cosmopolitan* (April 1960), but another woman could much less triumphantly refer to "The Day I Stopped Worrying About Tomorrow" (*Redbook*, May 1967). But this is as much a history of women beginning to write about their own MS as it is the story of the decay of the personal-triumph metaphor, unsustained as it was by further victories in war.

Through the efforts of the NMSS and its growing number of chapters, MS developed a public reputation. Helped by the solidarity of war and by the centralized nature of advertising and publishing immediately after the war, the Society's preferred images were widely disseminated. The isolation and hopelessness of many MS patients was diminished. Their families and other members of the local community stood a better chance of knowing something about the disease apart from a particular case. This was the basis for dissent as much as for uniform acceptance of imagery. Where previously MS was an act of diagnosis under the control of physicians, it now was an enemy to be fought using whatever means available.

Individuals in the United States could choose to ignore the MS definition that doctors were attempting to foist on them, and they could disagree with the picture of MS patients nationally promoted by the MS society. These departures from medical and advertising dogmas were themselves absorbed into publicity or remained local or private. As the population of those who knew they had MS grew, their demand for a simple cure became a force in itself, one that the MS society tried to represent and harness. But the society's commitment to careful medical research was at odds with the urgent wishes of patients. As government regulatory authorities came to decide on the release of medications, patient demands became a fourth component of public discourse on MS, often at odds with the medical researchers, the government and the MS society.

In 1942 the Soviet research team of Margulia, Soloviev and Choubladze isolated five strains of a virus they named E.H.A., after the French name for the disease from which the patients suffered: *encéphalomyélite humaine aigue* (acute human encephalomyelitis). As they reported to the English-reading world in 1946, one strain of this virus, called SV after the name of the patient from whom it was taken, was neutralized (deprived of infectiousness in animals) by the blood sera of people recovering from encephalomyelitis or with multiple sclerosis. Sera from people with other diseases of the central nervous system did not neutralize the virus. Choubladze and her colleagues reasoned that in the SV sera, they had a vaccine against demyelinating diseases, especially MS, because the sera must contain antibodies against the E.H.A. virus.

After the war, the "vaccine of Margoulis and Choubladze" went into production at the Metchnikoff Institute in Kharkoff. The brains of rats and mice infected with the SV strain of the virus were put into a liquid suspension treated with formalin to kill intrusive bacteria. The vaccine was distributed within the Soviet Union but also was made available for export. A manual of instructions for the administration of the treatment decreed two or three courses of subcutaneous injection of the vaccine, which could be repeated. Choubladze and others delivered papers on their tests at international pathology conferences (1956), giving the details of their further researches. They acknowledged that the E.H.A. virus resembled the rabies virus but added that there were striking differences between this virus and rabies in the pathology of the brain and in clinical symptoms.

The promotional effort was a success in reaching MS patients outside the Soviet Union. On July 13, 1956, the *New York Times* reported the USSR press charges that the United States had banned import of the vaccine after American MS victims had requested it. The Federal Drug Administration replied that there was insufficient information on the vaccine but added that both American and Swedish investigators had thrown doubt on the value of the treatment.

In the spring of 1957, Dr. R. S. Allison of Queen's University of Belfast, Northern Ireland, noted requests to obtain the vaccine for patients. Throughout 1958 the *British Medical Journal* printed exchanges between physicians presenting requests for their "anxious" patients and the Minister of Health, who was not sure the vaccine had the qualities claimed for it.

The minister cited an article by Dick, McKeown and Wilson (1958) reporting negative results of tests with the vaccine. "We have been unable to find that sera of patients in Northern Ireland with multiple sclerosis show any significant neutralization of the SV strain of E.H.A. virus." The team found that the virus samples supplied by the Soviet workers could not be differentiated from rabies virus. Demands for the Soviet MS vaccine diminished over the following years, although a rumor persisted that "the Russians have a cure for MS."

The MS vaccine episode was a minor one in the history of scientific posturing that made up the Cold War. In the history of MS, it did demonstrate the force that patient demand was beginning to exercise. Patient demand to import the drug caused an international trade incident. Feeling pressure to make the vaccine available through the national health plan, British health authorities supported scientific testing, which discredited the vaccine at least to the extent of denying it candidacy for inclusion in MS treatment provided. The U.S. drug authorities, also responding to tests, simply excluded the vaccine, which act the Soviets claimed was politically motivated. The would-be vaccine suppliers had attempted to sell their product to patients through rumor by appealing to mistrust of national and medical authorities. The doctors and MS societies, for their part, were willing to test the vaccine and discourage their patients from having it administered once its nature was discovered.

Other proposed treatments were more difficult to exclude. Hinton Jonez was a general practitioner in Tacoma, Washington, then a small town out of the New York–Chicago–Los Angeles ambit of specialists like Tracy Putnam. Yet Jonez gained a national reputation as a treater of MS and received patients from all over the country. He had developed a professional interest in allergy and was an early member of the American College of Allergists. For him, MS was the result of an allergic reaction causing the constriction of cerebral blood vessels and the resultant destruction of myelin through loss of nourishment. It was Rindfleisch's revision of Virchow's theory cast in terms of the experimental allergic encephalopathy research of the 1930s–40s.

Jonez had chosen to interpret the clinical trials of histamine as an MS treatment during 1942–44 as successful, and he practiced a regimen of intravenous histamine for the early cases together with an antispasmodic curare derivative (turbocurarine) for more progressed ones. Attention to diet, physical therapy and psychotherapy was also important to his system, which was more interdisciplinary than the single succeed-or-fail treatments of the specialists. He centered his practice on a Roman Catholic teaching hospital, St. Joseph's in Tacoma, though he placed no denominational restrictions on his patients. The Catholic background of the Mayo Clinic and its similar degree of geographic isolation in Rochester, Minnesota, suggest that Jonez's MS clinic was modeled in opposition to the cosmopolitan medical establishment. The emphasis on the then-abandoned (even by Mayo) histamine treatments cast Jonez in the role of a stubborn advocate for what was most effective for the patients, against the incomprehensible scientific pretensions of the established urban doctors. "Therapeutic nihilism" was a phrase Jonez also used.

The openness of Jonez's clinic and the use of broader therapies to restore the use of limbs and instill confidence in patients contributed to his success. It also gave him a poor reputation with the MS society and specialists. In 1950 Tracy Putnam replied to a woman whose mother was planning to go to the Tacoma clinic, telling her that the same treatment was available at many other clinics, that he and others had had "indifferent success" with it but that it was harmless (Talley 1995:55). The MS society, alert to potential deceit of patients, was less measured in its criticism.

Hundreds of MS and other central nervous system disease patients made their way to Tacoma between 1947 and 1953, when Jonez's death (October 11) closed the clinic. In his popular book *My Fight to Conquer Multiple Sclerosis*, "as told to" the professional writer Miriam Zeller Gross and published by the New York firm of Julian Messmer (1952), Jonez used the same metaphors as did the MS society to express his alternate campaign against the disease. Jonez described cases of patients who came to him after being mistreated by other practitioners. One woman had a hysterectomy because her doctor interpreted her MS symptoms as hysteria; others were simply told that they had nothing wrong with them or were suffering from a hopeless disease. Jonez's combination of therapies benefited all of these patients.

Books by individual physicians trumpeting the success of their idiosyncratic therapies are as old as medicine. There had been a number on cancer, tuberculosis and polio. Jonez's book was the first on MS, adopting the MS society's personalistic approach but embracing a therapy it did not approve. Jonez identified himself as a treating physician; his only research was to study the relative efficacy of his treatments. In a posthumously published paper (Jonez 1953), for instance, he described using eosinophil (leukocyte) determinations to measure the progress of histamine therapy. His career also countered the growing split between laboratory researchers and practitioners. Contemporaries like Putnam concentrated on laboratory experiments at one phase in their careers and then moved on to emphasize practice. In this way too, Jonez represented a perpetuation of an older medical career pattern in the public milieu. Like the folksy radio and newspaper doctors of his time, he was the country doctor who spoke through a microphone. He was the country doctor who signed on with New York publishers.

For all the conservatism of his manner and technique, Jonez was not retrograde in the treatments he advocated. Another component in his populism was an attempt to integrate treatments, in effect constructing a medical holism out of professionally separated therapeutic components. In the final paper in his series on MS (Jonez 1951), he wrote, "Psychotherapy ... plays the major role in all of our various approaches to the symptomatic treatment of these patients." Jonez explained that the entire central nervous system had originated embryologically from the same tissue layer and that both are subjected to the same allergic insults. Urticarial wheals caused by food allergy or emotion can expand on the skin or intestinal tract without hindrance, but when they occur inside the skull or spine, the result can be pressure that cuts off the blood supply and causes scar tissue and plaques. If the allergic reaction ceases soon enough, the pressure drops and there is a remission. In this way, Jonez linked the pathology of MS to allergic causes and supported the use of histamine for vasodilation therapy to reduce the pressure.

Obviously, prevention and long-range treatment lay in addressing the psychological underpinnings of allergy. After analyzing a large number of cases, Jonez reached the conclusion that a strong emotion triggers the first MS attack rather than the other way around, much as urticaria appears on the skin after emotional trauma. He gave a number of brief examples to illustrate the precipitating role of trauma: an engineering officer caught between decks during the war was paralyzed from the waist down and then experienced the remission and exacerbation cycle of MS; a priest going to the altar to be ordained suffered paralysis of the foot, stumbled and thereafter suffered MS; a girl paralyzed on the day before her wedding; "not a few first noticed symptoms of the disease during divorce proceedings or immediately after." By linking a causal complex of MS already embedded in the medical literature to blatant emotional states and declaring psychotherapy the main treatment supplemented by drugs, Jonez fashioned a simple explanation for the disease with a complex background. Anyone who had been subjected to a trauma might explain symptoms like those of MS in terms of the allergic reaction precipitated by that trauma. Jonez publicized, if not originated, a powerful popular explanation for a very old symptom set. With no technique for detecting the presence of plaques in the brains of the living, who could contradict the details of the theory?

By equating MS with allergic skin reactions, Jonez removed the hidden mystery and opened up contacts with therapeutic systems, diet and physical therapy, seldom used by orthodox physicians in his time. His MS complex helped establish a strain of MS representation that did not depend on physicians or the MS society. Despite the scientific references Jonez's therapy was a throwback to therapies used as early as d'Esté and used all along by people who did or did not know they had MS. In the early 1950s these therapies became specific to MS, whereas before they may simply have applied to all serious cases of persistent vertigo. People who were in effect silenced by the shame or uncertainty of their illness, or by the lack of access to forms of expression and a language of symbols, now were able to state their condition publicly, present their views on its cause whether in keeping with medical doctrine or not and bring forward therapies now specifically applied to MS. Jonez was one physician who attempted to take part in this general liberation of MS discourse from the control of the establishment physicians and the MS society.

Public MS discourse was reflecting a rapid diversification in MS research. The apparent antagonism between a "popular" body of opinion and medical or official doctrine was often the surfacing of a controversy, previously conducted among researchers, into the popular media. Research papers expressed findings, which the media reported in less technical terms, which then were adopted into the views of individuals, becoming a motive for the funding of more research and for further popular expression. This process contributed to the idea of MS as a mysterious and highly complex disease not yielding to known treatments. Jonez's return to histamine after it had been rejected by most neurologists was the harbinger of many other theoretical-therapeutic regimens that looked back to earlier research and treatments.

To maintain contact with the public of MS patients and their families, the growing medical research industry had to present its work in terms of simple catchphrases devoid of scientific ambiguity. Doctors seemed powerless and even confused when they tried to describe the scientific rationale for their endless inconclusive experiments. Statements like "MS is an allergic reaction" or "MS is due to pressure in the brain" or "sludged blood" made the scientists appear to be in control and a cure appear to be on the way. The need for publicity-oriented simplification could also yield concise statements not accurately reflecting the research that gave them birth. "Multiple Sclerosis Linked to Cosmic Rays," proclaimed *Science Digest* (December 1960) at a time when these dramatic "cosmic rays" were also being associated with cancers, birth defects and extraterrestrial activities. Even when the slogan version of a discovery was correct, the statement sounded more definite than the research itself provided. "Measles Antibodies Possible Clue to Multiple Sclerosis" (*Science News Letter*, January 12, 1963) was tentative-sounding, but "Multiple Sclerosis Linked to Chicken Pox Virus" (*Science News Letter*, April 3, 1965) gives the impression that the virus causes the disease. The multiplication of statements like this kept MS a mystery.

Awareness of MS among Americans remained dependent on personal contact with the disease either through having it oneself or through a friend or relative's affliction. The constant supply of articles in magazines telling of a musician's or an athlete's diagnosis and struggle depended on audience awareness of that person. Given the specialized interests of the popular audience, these people could not serve as surrogates for a general awareness of MS. Occasionally, a figure with MS would occupy national attention, as when Iran hostage Richard Queen was released from captivity due to his need for medical attention for MS. MS never had its FDR or Lou Gehrig. But then there are reasons to hope it never does.

Though the availability of information about the disease has increased with the general increase of information availability, it is still one item among many for all but those afflicted and their circles. Infectious diseases with much smaller numbers of victims capture popular imagination more readily than slow, indefinable MS. An outbreak of casualties among children infected with a virulent strain of E. coli bacteria garnered much more publicity than the story of a cluster of workers in a zinc plant all coming down with MS. As bacteria have given way to viruses as the villains of choice in news reports and science fiction, reports of virus epidemics in Africa make headlines while Africa itself is ignored. As an obscure disease with mostly obscure victims and not a dramatically virulent visualizable organism, MS is not suited to star status.

The amount of MS diagnosis leads to attempts to validate the disease in the most potent current categories. A recent subject search of viral diseases in the Marin County Library database turned up MS: the MS-virus links described in the press were enough to make MS a viral disease at least in that librarian's mind. Though MS is associated with viruses, MS is not associated with AIDS, yet physicians routinely test people with MS symptoms for HIV. Some potent categories just don't merge.

While research goes forward and concepts about MS attain tentative verification, transmission from the scientific media continues to depend on the drama and conciseness of the phrase. MS has become an "autoimmune disease" and, with the discovery of a set of predisposing genes, a "hereditary disease" for some people. This in turn allows it to be connected to other autoimmune or hereditary diseases and thus both inscribed in and circumscribed by the scientific effort. MS can then be like any of these other diseases.

As drug companies become major subsidizers of their own proprietary research on MS, another channel of refraction is opened quite close to the scientific source. An employment ad by Chiron (*San Francisco Chronicle*, October 27, 1996) boasts, among other accomplishments, that the company produced "the first effective treatment for multiple sclerosis" (a form of interferon). The chemical firm Pfizer, in an advertisement in *Scientific American* (November 1996), claims to be working on a cure for "congenital multiple sclerosis."

In the late 1970s, 77-year-old Dr. Ben J. Sheppard of Miami, Florida, offered treatments for MS and arthritis at his clinic. His PROven vaccine consisted primarily of snake venom harvested by a veteran snake collector. The treatments were inexpensive: $200 for a three-week course at the clinic and 100 injections to be taken at home. Patients' testimonials were quoted in articles in national magazines (*Newsweek*, December 1979), and more arrived from all over the country. Dr. Sheppard told a *Newsweek* reporter that he did not know how the snake venom worked, just that it did. Dr. Byron W. Waksman, the medical director of the NMSS (quoted in the same article), said that water would have the same effect on MS patients. Although Dr. Sheppard and his successors will always have business, MS remains public in this way.

14

The Prayers
of Vernon Olayos

Muz Olayos told me that her son Vernon had a beautiful voice. He played the guitar and sang for children in schools, at family gatherings and by himself in his room at the seminary where he was studying for the priesthood. On May 23, 1967, he wrote in the diary he had been keeping since the previous January. "Well, I discovered one thing, *once again*, I cannot come close to what I used to be able to do (e.g., I can just barely push a mop around my floor and I cannot play the guitar 1/421,367,589th as well as I used to (?), in other words I'm a complete *MESS*)." The last diary entry was in May. In June he was taken home from the seminary. The medical tests performed in the hospital indicated that he had multiple sclerosis. Vernon remained at home under his mother's care until his death by asphyxiation on November 20, 1967.

Muz found the diary among Vernon's school papers a year and a half later. She carefully edited his entries, eliminating pages of repetition and scrawl but not cutting out his torments, his account of attraction to a fellow seminarian and his very infrequent use of the word "shit." Muz commissioned the famed San Francisco printers Lawton and Alfred Kennedy to design and handset a book from the edited diary (Olayos 1971). The austerely attractive book has a gold Maltese cross embossed on its front cover. Its main title, *If I Should Die*, comes from a favorite children's prayer: "Now I lay me down to sleep / I pray the Lord, my soul to keep. / If I should die before I wake, / I pray the Lord my soul to take." The prayer is printed at the head of the dedication page.

A copy of the book resides in the History of Medicine Collection in the University of California–San Francisco Library. But Muz did not intend it to be a work on multiple sclerosis, and indeed there are no references at all to MS in Vernon's entries, only in the brief preface and the doctor's note at the end. Muz says she had scarcely heard of MS before she learned of the diagnosis.

Vernon wrote his entries as a chronicle of a spiritual struggle that affected his health and his ability to achieve his life's mission. His mother edited them accordingly. Her treasured reaction to the book was when a priest told her that seminarians at a retreat lined up to read the one copy available.

Muz and her family understood Vernon's tribulations as a spiritual struggle but more urgently as a matter of physical health that did not have to be accepted passively. The seminary authorities thought Vernon had a "nervous breakdown" and put him under the care of a spiritual adviser. Muz objected, arguing before the bishop that Vernon was better cared for at home. The published diary is dedicated to three medical doctors. No priest contributed to or is mentioned outside the text of the diary.

This diary marks a historic process of transition from a life within the context of a circumscribed religious community with its own categories of physical unease to a life within the broadly public, secular and scientific categories of disease. Diaries of spiritual grappling with physical decay have been written in the West since antiquity. Vernon's predecessors within this tradition were troubled by cancers, migraines, ulcers, hallucinations, interfering relatives and much more. MS was just another name for the particulars of a trial. Possibly others with MS, who didn't know they had MS and were not among people who could tell them so, wrote similar diaries 100 or 200 years ago. In the published form of Vernon's diary, for the first time the sufferer's diary genre converges with the name of multiple sclerosis. Medicine gives a name to the affliction that the person has been treating as a fault in his relation with divinity, with the world and with other humans. Stories we might have known as religious, social or political are subsumed beneath the label of MS.

Vernon's diary was preceded by the writings of d'Esté, Barbellion and all the pieces by and about people with MS, appearing in U.S. and European magazines starting in the late 1940s. Apart from these, Vernon's is the earliest of the nearly 100 personal MS accounts listed in this book's bibliography of autobiographies, biographies, novels, videos, studies and films. Though he was not writing with the knowledge that he had MS, his family's action to preserve his record marks the beginning of an autobiographical subgenre: the personal disease narrative focused on the ravages of MS.

This is primarily an American, English-language writing of MS history. It may be because the United States is the largest and most populous nation subject to high rates of MS and has a large publishing industry and a readership familiar with the disease. Vernon Olayos' diary seems to be the last published MS account written entirely in day-by-day form (as Barbellion's and d'Esté's also were) and the last one in which the author was not aware that he had MS while writing most or all of it (Barbellion knew close to the end). After this point, authors write the books because they know they have MS.

These recent books are as much a record of symptoms as the earlier ones were, but the writers now are conscious of MS, a medical condition, which in turn may be a symptom of some greater matter in their lives, possibly spiritual or moral — gender identity, profession, family relations, business or artistic dedication, to mention but a few.

The life stories of people with MS are the culmination of the long medical development of the MS concept. From the 1830s, when the first lithographic pictures appeared, to the present slow-motion MRI sequences of the changes in cerebral lesions available over the Internet, MS has become progressively known as an appearance of brain tissue. People who learn they have MS must absorb the presence of these invisible cellular abnormalities and work them into those body states that, they are told, are symptoms of the disease. MS narratives are attempts to absorb medically defined sensations into social and family life.

Until recent years there has not been a patient's history of MS to parallel the doctors' medical history. For the most part patients were isolated from each other and had their relation with the disease defined by the physicians and researchers who named both disease and patient. The medical history can claim that it is a universal history of discovering basic truths of the human body. The patient's history is the product of an environment with the leisure for self-reflection and writing. Cancer has been recognized for a very long time, but only recently, in Europe, America and Japan, have people set down the stories of their cancer sufferings. The same is true of polio, TB, herpes, AIDS and a variety of mental illnesses. Even conditions like chronic fatigue syndrome have their sufferers' tales in print. There is a large personal literature on anorexia.

One major difference between the early MS narratives (d'Esté, Barbellion, Olayos) and the more recent ones is the provision of advice. Vernon Olayos wrote his work as a spiritual diary, and it was framed by his family as a religious manual. Many of the books by people with MS published since then explicitly recommend coping strategies and treatments.

This literature grows out of another ancient practice: the advertisement of cure and advice. In the Temple of Aesculapius, the afflicted dreamed their cures and then became competent to assist others seeking relief. For centuries afterward, physicians advertised that they had healed themselves (and, of course, others) in proclaiming the value of their cures. On January 12, 1997, a national newspaper supplement magazine featured an article by a pathologist who had accidentally infected himself with HIV while performing an autopsy but who was able to banish the virus from his blood with disciplined medication. There has not been a comparable claim for MS.

Proclaiming *You Can Do It from a Wheelchair* (1973), Arlene Gilbert described her own debility due to MS paralysis and provided hints for performing tasks that invalids might not think possible. Her narrative was a pep talk aimed at people who might feel discouraged by the limitations their condition imposed on them. This "can-do" theme already was an American reworking of the Aesculapian narrative. Far from a dream, it was practical advice.

The previous year (1972) M. H. Greenblatt, in the brief book *Multiple Sclerosis and Me*, gave an account of his own diagnosis, with the stated intent of making the details of MS known to a wider public. A physicist employed by RCA before his debility made work difficult, Greenblatt devised and had built mechanisms to enable him to continue everyday life functions, like using the toilet and turning the pages of a book. He also commented on early events in his life — an accidental fall, difficulty with speech — which in retrospect seemed to be warning signs of the emergent disease.

Greenblatt's book was published by a Charles Thomas, a medical publisher specializing in technical and popular books on neurological conditions. In 1979 Thomas published another personal MS story, titled *Multiple Sclerosis: A Personal View* and written by a woman, Cynthia Birrer, but with an advisory intent that paralleled that of Greenblatt's earlier book.

Publishers with national distribution have issued very few of the MS autobiographies appearing since Vernon Olayos' diary. Most personal accounts of MS, like the Olayos book, have been self-published or published by small regional presses. The struggle against MS, the one element shared by all MS life stories, is not in itself sufficient to carry even a well-written manuscript to publication. MS patients and their families are not a large-enough market to support a book locally or nationwide without other interesting themes. The locally published accounts have a theme or quality that relates the MS battle to a specific set of interests or community of people.

Vernon Olayos' diary is a narrative of a man trying to reconcile his Roman Catholic faith with an affliction he can't name and does not understand. Other Christian responses to MS come in books by Opha Bingham (1985) and Patti Coghenour (1986). Bingham calls on her faith to keep her walking, whereas Coghenour, charismatic rather than evangelical, declares that she was miraculously healed of MS. The Reverend Charles Hunter and his wife, Frances, published through their own press a biography of Gene Lilly (1976), who was not healed of MS but who showed great faith during the trials of his illness.

Stories of endurance and of meeting death peacefully are outnumbered by the accounts of the miraculous healing of MS testified in articles that appear from time to time in the Christian press. MS has joined other afflictions as a specific opportunity to demonstrate divine workings in individual lives. The Christian healing narratives carry over to the testimonies of the efficacy of such popular therapies for MS (and arthritis) as systematically applied bee stings and injection of snake venom, whose practitioners often cite divine providence for creating these cures in nature and whose beneficiaries thank the Lord for the means to remission. Those skeptical of the direct or indirect divine cures invariably explain that MS can seem to cease because it is remitting-relapsing.

A Roman Catholic nun, Rita Klaus, has told of the unsettling effects of MS on her religious vocation (1993), and in a videotape (1995) she described her pilgrimage to Medjugorje in Croatia, where the Virgin Mary is believed to appear to (no longer) children. She does not look forward to a miraculous cure but rather to a strengthening of faith to help her live with the disease. She shares this reliance on faith with the evangelical Protestants who have written about their remissions from MS, and she also relies on the instrumentality of prayer as they do, though not on communal prayer. None of them reject medical treatment entirely, but they all believe that improvement is contingent on religious faith.

A Canadian Catholic with MS, Laurie Dennett, also undertook a pilgrimage, but to the medieval shrine of Santiago de Compostela in Spain. Her book (1987) is a lively travelogue of a woman who is curious about the place and the other pilgrims and who is more than half-hoping that she will gain some benefits, which in a way she does, though more from the investigations of travel than from any supernatural power of the shrine.

By far the greatest number of MS life stories, biographical or autobiographical, tell of the determination to live well in spite of the debilitating effects of the illness; they offer practical advice and counseling to the reader touched by MS. The MS sufferer might be portrayed (portraying him/herself) as an inspiration to others, like Vernon Olayos (or for that matter, Saint Lidwina), and as the practitioner of a technique — spiritual, psychological or material — for overcoming the disease. All published life stories contain some balance of these two elements.

John Pageler's autobiographical advice pamphlet is locally available at natural-food stores in central Florida. He summarizes its contents in the opening paragraph (Pageler 1986: 1): "ONE PATIENT, THE AUTHOR: John Pageler, that's me. ... I'm not a doctor nor a scientist. ... First, I speak from intimate, first-hand knowledge, because I am an MS patient myself. Secondly, I have kept the disease under control since it was diagnosed twenty-one years ago." Pageler chronicles his life from early fumbling attempts at sports to military service, more accidents and finally a loss of sight while driving, the last leading him to the MS diagnosis. He is disappointed by the failure of the medical doctors to offer him any hope and becomes slowly convinced by Dr. Roy Swank's theory that MS is caused by (high-fat) diet and can be cured by changing the foods consumed.

Swank cited the epidemiological studies comparing low-MS-rate fish-eaters with high-MS-rate dairy-users in Norway and recommended a low-fat mineral-enriched diet for MS patients. Pageler portrays the National MS Society membership in Portland as a group of defeatist invalids in contrast to Dr. Swank's followers, who are upbeat and free of the worst ravages of the disease. Despite his declared mistrust of people with academic credentials, he espouses Swank's approach due to its observable efficacy. Pageler briefly describes the main theories of MS causation, declaring that Swank and Horrobin's idea of unprocessed fat causing blood clots makes the most sense. "I have never met any patient who had gotten any medical treatment, orthodox or non-orthodox, from acupuncture to implant surgery, from cortisone injections to snake venom injections who felt they had long term benefits" (Pageler 1986:36).

Pageler emerges as a strong, honest, determined man who is the living example of his own therapeutic usage. He even built his health-food businesses on the dietary knowledge that came with his personal defeat of MS debility (if not of the disease itself). He gives his address and phone number and the times those with questions can call him. He refers to "the Lord" several times, but his visit to a church (the grandson of a Methodist clergyman, he did not follow organized religion) left him with a determination to find his own solution to the disease. He puts himself forward as the exemplar of an active approach, unlike the passive coping of the MS society members he mentions, but his life is similar to the others in advocating a means to reduce the effects of the disease. His vigor and certainty once he has proven the dietary approach are not unlike the conviction of the avowed Christian struggling against MS through prayer and pilgrimage.

Pageler takes an assertive role against MS by attempting to invent a solution of his own and letting others know that it works. This might even be called a "masculine" approach to MS life history. A magazine item like Jason Morin's "Rock Hard and in Remission from MS" (1994), describing a bodybuilder's success against the disease through exercise (and diet changes), is placed to address those with MS who identify themselves as bodybuilders. In *Spirit Makes a Man* (1978), the New York physician Joseph Panzarella, himself an MS patient, described the physical rehabilitation program he developed for people with disabilities like his. Panzarella's "spirit," both religious and personal, overcame the limitations of his condition to recover his manhood in helping others on the way to self-restoration.

But it is difficult to identify what elements of these life accounts are peculiarly masculine, since Pageler, Morin and Panzarella address both men and women. They may promote themselves as male exemplars, but their disease can affect anyone. *Runner's World* magazine printed an article (Kowalchik 1994) on Darlene Wojiski, an employee who was diagnosed with MS but who would not be discouraged from running competitively. The autobiography of Moira Griffin (1989) centers around her becoming aware of her physical deficiencies as she runs for exercise. She received training advice that enabled her to continue running while not making excessive demands of herself. Both the article and the book treat MS as a personal challenge to the individual who, with support, special exercise and dietary adjustments, is able to remain competitive.

Gender is a matter that MS history has developed but not confronted. The subject is in any reading of MS life stories, whether the writer intended to raise it or not. MS distribution has a gender bias, with women having the preponderance of afflictions. Once the statistics clearly gave women half as many again the number of cases as men, there was little attempt to explain the difference, perhaps because the biological differences had long been used to substantiate temperamental stereotypes.

Women, prone to "hysteria," many early physicians believed, would also be prone to MS. But Charcot and other students of hysteria thought that men were more likely to exhibit its symptoms. The earliest published MS autobiographies were written by men. It was only with the emergence of the MS societies that women's MS stories began to appear alongside those by men. Women now publish at least as many book-length MS autobiographies as men.

Writing about their MS has become a route to autobiography for women. It has for men as well, inspiring those who might not have told their stories to set them down. But women writers find MS an experience connected to other struggles of their lives, whereas men often treat it as a new challenge to be overcome.

Men are the preferred subject in fictional treatments of MS. Four fictional portrayals of people with MS in American writing (Hassler 1981; Milofsky 1981; Scoppetone 1982; Elkin 1993), by very different authors writing for different audiences, all show males afflicted with the disease. In David Milofsky's novel *Playing from Memory* (1981), the talented violinist Ben Seidler is paralyzed by MS at the peak of his career. A man coming down with MS is a dramatic reversal of fortune, one that male energy, however expressed, cannot overcome. Seidler's wife helps him to cope with his debility and live his life on new terms. In Jon Hassler's *The Love Hunter* (1981), the protagonist plots to murder his best friend, paralyzed with MS, ostensibly to put him out of his misery but perhaps in truth to claim his wife.

The only two fiction films I know of featuring people with MS center around women. The two films are the greatest imaginable contrast to each other. *Ich klage an* (1941) was produced in Nazi Germany as a propaganda piece promoting euthanasia. A doctor seeking a cure for MS gives his beautiful wife, who has developed the disease, a lethal injection rather than watch her degenerate into paralysis. The woman is portrayed as passive and grateful. In *Eden* (1996), the afflicted woman is the wife of a rigid prep school teacher. Studying mysticism, she drifts off further and further into a dreamworld until, lying in a coma, she gets to decide to live when her husband disconnects her life-support respirator.

Of these fictional accounts, the only one by a writer himself suffering from MS (Elkin 1993) in fact concerns the relationship between a college professor with a debilitating neurological condition and his wife, who leaves him at a critical stage in his life ("Her Sense of Timing") after having been a tolerant caregiver for a long time. The professor goes on with his routines in her absence, which seems to promote some independence for him as well. This rare fictional portrayal of relations in a couple dealing with the chronic disease of one emphasizes the same need to break away from dependencies that women themselves emphasize in their autobiographical accounts. In this account, the woman's move out of the relationship precipitates the man's grudging self-sufficiency.

Couples, the interplay between men and women, are the arena in which the effects of MS diagnosis and changing debility are most fully played out. Many autobiographies of MS people and fictions about them are about relations in couples and with family members of the opposite sex. The pressure of MS gives an edge to the mingled, but not always contrary, forces of independence and dependency needs. David Milofsky's Ben Seidler needs the support of his wife, Dory, to go on with his life amid the devastations of MS.

John and Alice Johnson, a Florida couple, have published two books on *their* struggle with John's multiple sclerosis (which they name "mysterious stranger," yet another mysterious MS) and with Alice's bulimia. Their first book was written by each in alternate chapters, giving the most balanced couple view of life with MS in all the writings. But here the couple can aid each other.

By contrast and in complement, there is Marion Deutsche Cohen's *Dirty Details: The Days and Nights of a Well Spouse* (1996), which is in the voice of a woman as caregiver for a husband afflicted with MS. When Stanley Elkin portrayed a couple broken up by a wife's decision to go her own way, he did not write in the wife's voice, nor have any of the other fiction and autobiographical writers who acknowledge woman caregivers. Cohen asserts the identity of the other, well person in an MS relationship and shows that the role is far from pleasant. In doing so, she fills in the other half of the couple.

Women often volunteer for and/or are relegated to caregiver roles in many societies. Much of the literature written about males with MS places the woman herself in the background while keeping in the foreground her role in the man's particular struggle. Joseph Panzarella, M. H. Greenblatt and John Pageler thank their wives, but as wives, the women do not have much of a personality other than that of a supportive spouse. Cohen's decision to provide care is not a reflex of her position but is the result of changing emotions. She is an independent person taking up the caregiver role and not consumed by it.

The condition of women as caregivers becomes yet more complex when the ailing other person is a mother or daughter. A mother's role in her daughter's development gives any chronic illness a painful twist for both (Derricotte 1992). Maturation is compromised as childish dependencies threaten to reassert themselves. Marilee Horton simply titled her memoir of her mother's illness *Dear Momma, Please Don't Die* (1979). In her diary of her daughter's confinement in a nursing home, Nellie Collar Anson (1992) sounded a mother's frustration at not being able to care for her child at home or assure her of good care in an institution.

When women write their own MS lives, they reflect on these patterns of dependence and independence. Janet Lee James, a young disc jockey at a Pittsburgh radio station, breaks up with her partner in the aftermath of an MS diagnosis; he takes up a long-planned cross-country trip, and she heads for Alaska and new relationships. Her heartfelt autobiography (1993) follows her life in the open landscape, on the open sea and in the closed cabins of the north. I have known others without the temperature needs who went from the urban north to escape in the farther north. But James' MS gives her version of this quest for independence while maintaining human relations a new poignancy. In the final pages, she writes of her hope for a cure.

Another woman with MS struggling for independence, and seeking it eventually in Alaska, was Faye Morgan. Her autobiographical novel (recalling in its title an early MS diagnostic test) *Riding the Gold Curve* (1994), tells how MS (and chemistry courses) defeated her aspirations to become a doctor. She was able to become a public health nurse and, battling to overcome the influence of her possessive brother, traveled from her home in Texas to Kansas and Alaska, to work with migrant laborers.

If James and Morgan are powerfully determined to win and keep independence, Barbara Webster is analytical and approaching anger. Her *All of a Piece* (1989) tends to dismay readers, both with MS and not. An anthropology graduate, she contrasted the accommodating response to her disability in an Egyptian village with the callous dismissal she received in public places in the United States. She enters a brief against the effects that American self-reliance and individualism have on the treatment of those who can't keep up with the pace.

These lives all write short histories of MS in our time and place. Themes and concerns that might rise up in any life — career, well-being, vital personal relationships — are all magnified by the gesture of MS. No longer silent, they add their sentences to the long history of MS, which by their addition is no longer a matter of case histories, tissue samples and pathogens. With them the tissue samples once again have a name.

Recently while I was seated on a mass-transit train, an elderly woman stood up in the car and, holding before her a plastic card most would recognize as a disabled ID card, declared that she had multiple sclerosis and that her HMO would not admit her unless she paid a $20 fee. During the same week a social activist crippled by MS was struck by a van while crossing a major intersection in her wheelchair. Neither of these events was caused directly by MS, but neither would have occurred if it weren't present. And both events bring forth elements in MS history that are of the moment — the state of the elderly, the role of HMOs, the behavior of traffic — and of all time. This, in the end, is what I mean by the history of MS: Lives written and unwritten that are of the moment and for all time.

Appendix: List of Attempted MS Treatments

*Presence in this list does not connote success,
only that the treatment has been tried.*

ACTH (adrenocorticotrophic
  hormone)
BAL
bee stings (apitherapy)
betahistinedimesilate
beta-interferon
carbamazepine (Tugretol)
diet changes
d-tubocararine
electrical stimulation (galvanic/
  faradic)
estrogen
evening primrose oil (colichinine)
exercise
fever therapy (malarial)
histamine

horseback riding
hyperbaric oxygen
insulin
laminectomy
penicillamine
phenytoin
Purves-Stewart vaccine
Shubladze vaccine
spinal cord stimulation
steroids
suboccipital puncture
temperature (hot/cold baths)
tolbutamide
vasodilation (CO_2)
vitamins

Bibliography

Autobiographies, Biographies,
Novels, Videos, Studies and Films

Anson, Nellie Collar. 1992. *Shattered Dreams: A Nursing Home Nightmare, a True Story from a Mother's Diary. The Gripping Account of Her Daughter's Battle for Life and the Day-to-Day Horror of Confinement in a Modern Nursing Home.* Houston, Tex.: Larksdale. [A rare MS diary by a parent and caregiver.]

Arrabal, Fernando. 1987. *The Compass Stone.* New York: Grove Press.

Atwood, Dave. 1986. *Tomorrow Is a Better Day.* New York: Vantage Press.

Austin, Bill. 1979. *And Stumbled on a Morning.* Wheaton, Ill.: Tyndale House. [Good title: a Baptist minister's story of his MS.]

Baer, Judy. 1995. *Silent Thief.* Minneapolis, Minn.: Bethany House Publishers. [Juvenile Christian novel in a series: family copes with mother's MS with a renewal of faith.]

Barbellion, Wilhelm Nero Pilate [Bruce Frederick Cummings]. [1919] 1984. *The Journal of a Disappointed Man; and, A Last Diary.* London: Hogarth Press. [A recent edition of the deliberately literary work by a young British naturalist asserting his life force against the sapping disease.]

_____. 1973. *Enjoying Life and Other Literary Remains.* N.Y.: Gordon Press.

Beach, Barbara. 1976. *MS and Us: An Autobiography.* Hicksville, New York: Exposition Press, 1976.

Besyk, Patti Coughenour, with Cliff Dudley. 1986. *By His Stripes: Healed of MS.* Green Forest, Ariz.: New Leaf Press.

Bingham, Opha, with Robert E. Bingham. 1985. *One Step More, Lord!* Nashville, Tenn.: Broadman Press.

Birrer, Cynthia. 1979. *Multiple Sclerosis: A Personal View.* Springfield, Ill.: Thomas.

Bjork, Ray O. 1978. *Multiple Sclerosis and How I Live with It.* Phoenix, Ariz.: Birchbark Press. [93-page inspirational essay.]

Bourgeois, Verne Warren. 1995. *Persons: What Philosophers Are Saying About You.* Waterloo, Ontario: Wilfred Laurier University Press.

Brack, Joyce. 1981. *One Thing for Tomorrow: A Woman's Personal Struggle with MS.* Saskatoon, Saskatchewan: Western Producers Prairie Books.

Breaten, Karstin. 1975. *Takk for ener dag: Tanker i rollestollen* [*Thanks for Another Day: Thoughts and Reflections*]. Oslo: Luther.

Brenneman, Helen Good. 1975. *Learning to Cope.* Scottdale, Pa.: Herald Press.

Breslow, Rachelle. 1992. *Who Said So? A Woman's Journey of Self-Discovery and Triumph Over Multiple Sclerosis.* Berkeley, Calif.: Celestial Arts.

Brewster, Barbara. 1992. *Journey to Wholeness: When the Risk to Remain Tight in Bed Was More Painful Than the Risk It Took to Bloom.* Rutland, Ore.: Four Winds.

Brown, J. 1984. One man's experience with multiple sclerosis. In Simons 1984:21–29. [A New Zealand man whose lack of athletic prowess isolated him from his compatriots, and whose marriage is breaking up because of misdiagnosis as spinal tumor, becomes a teacher, then a journalist and an unofficial "stirrer" on behalf of MS people. "When the subtle cloud of tiredness and lethargy creeps over us, it seems so much easier to curl up like a well-fed cat and let life flow over us. That is exactly what it will do if that is your reaction." See Brewster 1992.]

Burnfield, Alexander. 1985. *MS: A Personal Exploration.* Souvenir Press.

Burstein (MacFarlane), Ellen, with Patricia Burstein. 1994. *Legwork: An Inspiring Journey Through a Chronic Illness.* New York: Charles Scribner's Sons. [Investigative reporter survives the decline of her marriage and the fraudulent treatment of a doctor with an exercise cure for MS.]

Ceccarelli, Marcello. 1976. *Viaggio provisorio: Breve storia di un uomo, della sui sclerosi a placche e di un esperimento finora mal riuscito* [*Tentative Voyage: Brief History of a Man, of His Multiple Sclerosis and of an Experiment Finally Unsuccessful*]. Bologna: Zanichelli. [An astronomer with MS.]

Chesto, Kathleen O. 1990. *Risking Hope: Fragile Faith in the Healing Process.* Kansas City, Mo.: Sheed and Ward, 1990.

Citino, David. 1990. *The Discipline: New and Selected Poems.* Columbus: Ohio State University Press.

Cohen, Marion Deutsche. 1996. *Dirty Details: The Days and Nights of a Well Spouse.* Philadelphia, Pa.: Temple University Press.

Cousins, Norman. 1979. *Anatomy of an Illness as Perceived by the Patient: Reflections on Healing and Regeneration.* New York: W. W. Norton. [Author's overcoming ankylosing spondylitis, not MS, but an inspiring work and quite influential.]

Davoud, Nicole. 1985. *Where Do I Go from Here? The Autobiography of a Remarkable Woman.* London: Piatkus.

Dean, Arline. 1995. *Multiple Sclerosis: The Unseen Enemy*. New York: Carlton Press. [Very brief, chatty life story by a woman with fairly mild MS, revealing how this unseen enemy can affect relationships with others.]

Delury, George E. 1997. *But What If She Wants to Die? A Husband's Diary*. New York: Birch Lane Press. [A caregiver's account of administering the ultimate care to (or murdering, depending on your view) his MS-afflicted wife.]

Dennett, Laurie. 1987. *A Hug for the Apostle*. Toronto: Macmillan of Canada. [Canadian woman with MS on a pilgrimage to Santiago de Compostela in Spain.]

Derricotte, Camille Ribera. 1992. "Daughters' Relative Development: The Effect of Having a Mother with MS" (project based upon independent interviews). Master's thesis, Smith College School of Social Work, Northampton, Mass.

Doherty, James. 1988. *It's Never the Same: A Priest's Struggle with MS*. Dublin: Irish Books and Media.

Edelman, Gerald. 1990. "How I Became Interested in Multiple Sclerosis." *Tikkun* 8:25–32.

Elkin, Stanley. 1993. *Van Gogh's Room at Arles*. New York: Simon and Schuster. [A collection of three stories by the American novelist who died in 1994; the protagonist of "Her Sense of Timing," a college professor debilitated by a neurological disease, must cope with his wife's inopportune departure.]

_____. 1994. "Out of One's Tree." In *The Best American Essays 1994*, ed. Tracy Kidder, pp. 92–109. Boston: Houghton-Mifflin. [To put it plainly: about the author's treatment with the drug Prednisone. "Because a sidebar of the loony, whacko condition is what it does to time ... being out of one's tree melts your watch like a Dali."]

Flood, Allan. 1993. *Perfect Misfortune: A Guide to Hope, Healing and Happiness During Personal Crisis*. Bend, Ore.: Pugrose Publications. [One of many books to address people with conditions like MS.]

Gettins, James. 1992. *The Door Is Always Open*. Boise, Idaho: Pathways Press.

Gilbert, Arlene. 1973. *You Can Do It from a Wheelchair*. New Rochelle, N.Y.: Arlington House. [Advice and encouragement for the disabled from a woman with MS.]

Ginther, John Robert. 1978. *But You Look So Well*. Chicago: Nelson Hall. [Chicago educator stricken with MS and not told of his condition for some years.]

Greenblatt, M. H. 1972. *Multiple Sclerosis and Me*. Springfield, Ill.: Thomas. [MIT physicist with MS exploring its possible origins in his life and describing devices he invented to make his work easier.]

[Greenhaven Press]. 1981. *Linda: A Victim of Multiple Sclerosis*. St. Paul, Minn.: Greenhaven Press. [Cassette tape — Insight series.]

Griffin, Moira. 1989. *Going the Distance: Living a Full Life with Multiple Sclerosis and Other Debilitating Diseases.* New York: Dutton.

Hassler, Jon. 1981. *The Love Hunter.* New York: Morrow. [Chris Mackensie plots to stage a hunting accident and kill his friend Larry Quinn, dying of MS. Chris hopes that Larry's wife and caregiver, Rachel, will then become available to him. It does work out that way, but not exactly as he had planned it.]

Hayes, James P. 1992. *MS'ing in Action.* N.p.: J. Hayes. [Jokes and cartoons with an MS-relieving theme.]

Herzen, Phyllis. 1982. *The Mustard Seed and Me.* N.p. [A manuscript deposited in the Spokane, Washington, public library.]

Hirsch, Ernest A. 1977. *Starting Over: The Autobiographical Account of a Psychologist's Experience with Multiple Sclerosis.* North Quincy, Mass.: Christopher Publishing House.

Hogan, Janis M. 1992. *In Spite of Everything.* [Tucson, Ariz.]: J. M. Hogan.

Horner, Bill. 1992. *The Last Dance Is Mine.* Montreal: Optimum Publishing International. [Canadian miner with MS.]

Horton, Marilee. 1979. *Dear Momma, Please Don't Die.* Nashville, Tenn.: Thomas Nelson. [Christian reflections on a mother's MS and clinical depression.]

Hunter, Charles, and Frances Hunter. 1976. *Don't Limit God: The Story of Gene Lilly.* Houston, Tex.: Hunter Ministries Press.

Huysmans, Joris Karl. 1979. *Saint Lydwine of Schiedam.* Trans. Agnes Hastings. Rockford, Ill.: TAN Books and Publishers.

Inglethorpe, Joy. 1989. *The Hope Merchants.* Johannesburg, South Africa: Hippogriff Press.

James, Janet Lee. 1993. *One Particular Harbor.* Chicago: Noble Press. [Fine narrative of a young disc jockey's MS diagnosis and her wanderings to Alaska and the Philippines, where she hoped for a cure from a massage healer.]

James, Martin. 1994. *Up Against It.* Marlborough, Wiltshire: Crowood Press. [British fisherman with MS.]

Johnson, John, and Alice Johnson. 1995. *Mysterious Stranger: A Couple's Courageous 40-Year Battle with Multiple Sclerosis.* Miami: Mal-Jonal Reading.
_____. 1996. *Mysterious Stranger Abroad.* Miami: Mal-Jonal Reading.

Key, Donald. n.d. *Future Unknown: A Family's Fight Against MS.* [Manuscript deposited in University of Michigan Library, 103 pp.]

King, Sylvia. 1975. *In Memoriam: Sylvia King.* London: Disablement Income Group.

Klaus, Rita. 1993. *Rita's Story.* Orleans, Mass.: Paraclete Press.
_____. 1995. *The Gift of Life.* Marian Press. [A 29-minute videotape on Rita Klaus and her pilgrimage to Medjugorje.]

Kowalchik, Claire. 1994. "The Nerve to Run." *Runner's World* 29, 11 (November): 23. [On Darlene Wojiski, employee of the magazine, who keeps up her running in spite of MS.]

Kuhlman, Kathryn. 1975. *Never Too Late.* Minneapolis, Minn.: Bethany Fellowship.

Kvaale, Kathy D. 1996. *I'm Not Drunk, I'm Not Crazy, Well Maybe a Little Nuts: Turning a Little Light on MS.* Fargo, N.D.: W.G. Writing.

Larouche-Thibault, Monique. 1988. *Un Amour comme le notre* [*A Love Like Ours*]. Montreal: Libre Expression.

Lishman, Alwyn. 1978. *Organic Psychiatry: The Psychological Consequences of Cerebral Disorder.* Oxford: Blackwell Sciences. [Multiple sclerosis, pp. 799–813, reviews the literature on the psychiatry of MS, describing the kinds of mental changes (euphoria, depression, intellectual impairment) found to be common in people with the disease.]

Loder, Cari. *Standing in the Sun.* [Rock journalist who earlier wrote about the singer Ricki Lake, who has MS, here tells of her discovery that a soft drink together with a drug cured her own MS.]

Lowry, Florence. 1984. One woman's experience with multiple sclerosis. In Simons 1984:30–35. [A singer diagnosed with MS on the eve of her wedding at age 20 briefly describes her changing psychological states, refers to the "skimpy mumbo-jumbo of the medical texts" and understandably wishes that her husband, instead of becoming national president of the Multiple Sclerosis Society, could be home with her more often.]

MacDougall, Roger. 1980. *My Fight Against Multiple Sclerosis.* Madison, Ohio: Regenics. [A 40-page pamphlet describing MacDougall's success overcoming the effects of MS through a very-low-fat diet.]

MacKarrel, Peter. 1990. "Interior Journey and Beyond: An Artist's View of Optic Neuritis." In *Optic Neuritis,* ed. R. F. Plant and H. E. Armstrong. Cambridge: Cambridge University Press. [Beautifully illustrated account of an artist's visions due to his disease.]

Mairs, Nancy. 1989. *Remembering the Bone House: An Erotics of Place and Space.* Perennial.

_____. 1993. *Ordinary Time: Cycles in Marriage, Faith, and Renewal.* Boston: Beacon.

_____. 1997. *Waist-high in the World: Life Among the Non-Disabled.* Boston: Beacon.

Medaer, R. 1979. "Does the History of Multiple Sclerosis Go Back as Far as the 14th Century?" *Acta Neurologica Scandinavica* 60:189–92.

Menninger, Dieter. 1978. *Beleugt uns nicht* [*Don't Lie to Us*]. Stuttgart: Kreuz Verlag.

Michael, Peter Paul. 1981. *Multiple Sclerosis: A Dragon with a Hundred Heads.* Port Washington, N.Y.: Ashley Books.

Moore, Sharon. 1995. *A Determined Spirit.* Shippensburg, Pa.: Destiny Image Press.

Morgan, Faye. 1994. *Riding the Gold Curve.* Lubbock: Texas Tech University Press. [Novel based on the author's own life story of her attempts to gain a medical education in spite of MS and her work as a nurse with migrant farm laborers and Alaska natives.]

Morin, Jason. 1994. "Rock Hard and in Remission from MS." *Muscle and Fitness* 55, 11 (November): 18.

Mortensson, Charlotte. 1996. "If My Life Becomes Unbearable I'll Kill Myself." *Prima.* May: 28.

Multiple Sclerosis Patients from Columbiana, Mahoning and Trumbull Counties, Ohio. 1984. *Recollections: Written for Newly Diagnosed Multiple Sclerosis Patients.* Youngstown, Ohio: Greater Youngstown Center of the Northeast Chapter of the National Multiple Sclerosis Society.

Mythen, John, et al. 1990. *Claude MSing Around: Fighting Against Multiple Sclerosis.* Seattle: Gordon Soules Books.

Nesbit, Betty. 1970. *The Day the Summer Ended.* London: Hodder and Stoughton. [Possibly the earliest published MS life.]

Olayos, Vernon Paine. 1971. *If I Should Die: The Diary of Vernon P. Olayos, edited by Dorothy Olayos.* San Rafael, Calif.: Lawton and Alfred Kennedy. [A young seminarian's diary as he struggles with his faith and, it turned out, acute MS.]

Ottenberg, Miriam. 1978. *The Pursuit of Hope.* New York: Rawson Associates Publishers.

Pageler, John. 1986. *New Hope, Real Help for Those Who Have Multiple Sclerosis.* Brandon, Fla.: The author. [By a former military man and health-food store operator who gained control of his MS through diet.]

Panzarella, Joseph, with Glenn D. Kittler. 1978. *Spirit Makes a Man.* Garden City, N.Y.: Doubleday. [A doctor is diagnosed with MS and establishes a rehabilitation clinic for patients with neurological disorders.]

Pawel, Ernst. 1995. *The Poet Dying: Heinrich Heine's Last Years in Paris.* New York: Farrar, Straus and Giroux.

Pekannen, John. 1998. "A Champion's Vow." *Reader's Digest,* February, 76–83. [Young Sarah Warnock's debility from MS and her courageous comeback.]

Perry, Sarah. 1994. *Living with Multiple Sclerosis: Stories of Coping and Personal Adaptation.* London: Avebury Press.

President's Committee on Employment of the Handicapped. 1984. *At Work: Profiles of People with Multiple Sclerosis.* Washington, D.C.: Government Printing Office.

[Project Rembrandt X]. 1993. *The Captive Will: An Exhibit of Works by 31 Artists with Multiple Sclerosis.* Pomegranate.

Pruet, Ronald Burton, and Myra Sue Pruet. 1976. *Run from the Pale Pony: Coping with Chronic Illness.* Grand Rapids, Mich.: Baker Book.

Queen, Richard, with Patricia Hass. 1981. *Inside and Out: Hostage to Iran,*

Hostage to Myself. New York: Putnam. [Taken hostage during the 1979 Iranian revolution, U.S. Consular Service employee Richard Queen was eventually released from his captivity due to an MS debility; not an MS autobiography so much as a crisis story in which MS played a role, with a little commentary on the attitudes of his captors and his reception in the United States.]

Reed, Sue, with Juanita Yates. 1990. *Journey of a Soul, in an MS Body.* Chicago: Avalus Press.

Robinson, Ian. 1988. *Multiple Sclerosis.* London: Routledge. [Experience of Illness series.]

_____. 1990. Personal narrative, social character and medical courses: Analysis of life trajectories in autobiographies of people with multiple sclerosis. *Social Science and Medicine* v. 30, n. 4 (June 1): 173 (Special Issue: Qualitative Research on Chronic Illness). [Analysis of life stories requested from members of an MS self-help group. "The particularly vigorous and positive approach that many people with multiple sclerosis take in attempting to achieve personal control over the effects of the disease is well demonstrated in many of the life stories considered here."]

Rodger, James. n.d. *MS: The Silent One.* [University of Michigan Library manuscript, 60 pp.]

Rubinstein, Renate. 1988. *Take It and Leave It.* Trans. from the Dutch by Karin Fierke and Aad Jensen. New York: M. Boyars.

Scoppetone, Sandra. 1982. *Long Time Between Kisses.* New York: Bantam. [Seventeen-year-old Billie James dyes her hair purple and falls in love with twenty-one-year-old Robert Mitchell, who has MS and is on crutches, but is it terminal?]

Shelly, Elaine. 1994. "The Years in Between." In *Life Notes: Personal Writings by Contemporary Black Women,* ed. Patricia Bell-Scott, pp. 281–99. New York: W. W. Norton. [Elaine Shelly's diary of her diagnosis of and coping with MS.]

Simons, Aart T. 1984. *Multiple Sclerosis: Psychosocial Aspects.* London: Heinemann Medical Books.

Smirnow, Eric, ed. 1993. *The MS Autobiography Book: An Anthology of Autobiographical Prose and Verse Written by Persons Who Have Multiple Sclerosis.* Cedaredge, Colo.: Special Computer Press.

Snider, Ron. 1995. *Saga: One Man's Battle with MS.* Kearney, Nebr.: Morris Publishing.

Spencer, Donald G. 1993. *A Unique Perception.* Pittsburgh, Pa.: Dorrance Press.

Sternberg, Nathalie. 1990[?]. *One Banana, Two Banana.* New York: New Day Films. [32-minute video about Lynne Sternberg, housewife with MS.]

Strasheim, Linda Light, with Evelyn Bence. 1985. *Something Beautiful*. Grand
    Rapids, Mich.: Zondervan Publishing House.
Topf, Linda Noble, with Hal Zina Bennett. 1995. *You Are Not Your Illness:
    Seven Principles for Meeting the Challenge of Illness*. New York: Simon and
    Schuster.
Walsh, Anthony, and Patricia Ann Walsh. 1989. "Love, Self-Esteem and Mul-
    tiple Sclerosis." *Social Science and Medicine* 29, 7:793–98. [By question-
    naires administered to 135 MS patients in southern Idaho, the authors
    found that "love was the most powerful predictor of self-esteem, followed
    by attitude stage, number of years since diagnosis, social class, and phys-
    ical restriction."]
Webster, Barbara. 1989. *All of a Piece: A Life with Multiple Sclerosis*. Baltimore:
    Johns Hopkins University Press. [Anthropology student with MS com-
    pares attitudes toward chronic disease in different cultures.]

Two Films About Multiple Sclerosis

Ich klage an (*I Cry Out*). (Film premier, Venice 1941.) Screenplay by Her-
    mann Schweninger, directed by Wolfgang Liebeneiner. A woman
    with MS is given a lethal dose of medication by her physician husband,
    who has sought a cure. She is contrasted with a child left alive but blind
    and deaf by meningitis. The film was made in close collaboration with
    the German führer's office. "Euthanasia" could not be mentioned in
    reviews.
Eden. Screenplay and directed by Howard Goldberg (shown at Mill Valley Film
    Festival, Oct. 6, 1996). A 29-year-old 1960s housewife with two children
    begins to astral project. She wears a legbrace, and we eventually learn she
    has MS. Her husband is a strict disciplinarian at the prep school where
    he teaches. He does not want her to teach, though she can. And he rides
    a gifted proto-hippie student who loves his wife. She helps the student
    with his studies but begins to spend more and more time away, goes into
    a coma and only comes back to be with her family when the husband dis-
    connects the respirator and gives her the opportunity to *choose*, as the wise
    old family doctor had suggested. Responding to questions afterward,
    Goldberg (his producer in shadows) maintained that the plot just came
    to him but that the woman character was inspired by a girl, with polio,
    on whom he had a crush in high school. In answer to my question, Gold-
    berg said that he chose MS because it is unpredictable and relapses-
    remits. MS references to ACTH treatment and medical bewilderment are
    accurate for the time.

General References

Acheson, E. D. 1972. "The Epidemiology of Multiple Sclerosis." In McAlpine, Lumsden and Acheson 1972:1–80.

Adams, A. 1989. "Was There a Multiple Sclerosis Epidemic in Kenya?" *East African Medical Journal* 66:503–6.

Adams, D. K. 1921. "The Cerebro-Spinal Fluid in Disseminated Sclerosis." *Lancet* 1:420–22.

Adams, F. 1856. *The Extant Works of Aretaeus the Cappadocian.* London: Bell and Underwood.

Allison, R. S. 1931. "Disseminated Sclerosis in North Wales." *Brain* 53:391–430.

Alter, Milton. 1962. "Multiple Sclerosis in the Negro." *Archives of Neurology* 7:83–92.

_____, and M. Harshe. 1975. "Racial Predilection in Multiple Sclerosis." *Journal of Neurology* 210:1–27.

_____, U. Leibowitz and J. Speer. 1966. "Risk of Multiple Sclerosis Related to Age at Immigration to Israel." *Archives of Neurology* 15:234–46.

_____, G. T. Sawyer and K. Latham. 1970. "The Frequency of Diabetes Mellitus in the Families of Patients with Multiple Sclerosis." *Neurology* 20:619–26.

_____, and John F. Kurtzke, eds. 1968. *Epidemiology of Multiple Sclerosis.* Springfield, Ill.: C.C. Thomas.

Althaus, Julius. 1878. *Diseases of the Nervous System.* New York: G.P. Putnam's Sons.

Aly, Götz, Peter Chroust, and Christian Pross. 1994. *Cleansing the Fatherland: Nazi Medicine and Racial Hygiene.* Trans. Belinda Cooper. Baltimore: Johns Hopkins University Press.

Baasch, E. 1966. Theoretische Überlegungen zur Ätiologie der Sclerosis multiplex: Die Multiple Sklerose eine Quicksilberallergie? *Schweize Archiv der Neurologie, Neurochirurgie und Psychiatrie* 98:1–37.

Babinski, Joseph. 1934. *Oeuvre scientifique.* Paris: Masson et Cie.

Baer, R. L., and M. B. Sulzberger. 1939. "Role of Allergy in Multiple Sclerosis." *Archives of Neurology and Psychiatry* 42:837.

Barbeau, Andre. 1958. "The Understanding of Involuntary Movements: An Historical Approach." *Journal of Nervous and Mental Disease* 127:469–89.

Barbour, Alan. 1996. *Lyme Disease: The Cause, the Cure, the Controversy.* Baltimore: Johns Hopkins University Press.

Barlow, J. 1960. "Correlation of the Geographic Distribution of Multiple Sclerosis with Cosmic Ray Intensities." *Acta Scandinavica Neurologica* 35 (Supplement 147):108–30.

Barnard, J. E. 1925. "The Microscopical Examination of Filtrable Viruses." *Lancet* 2:117–20.

Beckstead, Robert. 1996. *Survey of Medical Neuroscience.* New York: Springer-Verlag.

Behan, Peter O., and Wilhelmina Behan. 1982. "Sir Robert Carswell: Scotland's Pioneer Pathologist." In Rose and Bynum 1982:273–92.

Behring, Emil Adolf von, and Shibasaburo Kitasato. 1890. "Über das Zustandekommen der Diphtherie-Immunität und der Tetanus-Immunität bei Thieren." *Deutsche Medizinische Wochenschrift* 16:1113–14, 1145–48.

Bick, Katherine, Luigi Amaducci, and Giancarlo Pepeu, eds. 1987. *The Early Story of Alzheimer's Disease.* New York: Raven Press.

Bing, R., and H. Reese. 1926. "Die multiple Sklerose in der Nordwestschweiz" (Kantone Basel, Solothurn, Aargau, Luzern). *Schweiz Medizinische Wochenschrift* 56:30–34.

Bishop, D. Timothy, Catherine Faulk, and Jean McCluer, eds. 1987. *Genetic Epidemiology: Applications and Comparison of Methods.* New York: Liss.

Black, Kathryn. 1996. *In the Shadow of Polio: A Personal and Social History.* Reading, Mass.: Addison-Wesley.

Bradley, W. G., and C. W. M. Whitty. 1968. "Acute Optic Neuritis: Prognosis for the Development of Multiple Sclerosis." *Journal of Neurology, Neurosurgery and Psychiatry* 31:10–15.

Brain, W. Russell. 1940. *Diseases of the Central Nervous System.* London: Oxford University Press.

Bramwell, Byrom. 1904. "On Disseminated Sclerosis, with Special Reference to the Frequency and Etiology of the Disease." *Clinical Studies: A Quarterly Journal of Clinical Medicine,* new series, 2:193–210.

Brickner, R. M., and C. R. Franklin. 1944. "Visible Retinal Arteriolar Spasm Associated with Multiple Sclerosis." *Archives of Neurology and Psychiatry* 51:573–81.

Bright, Richard. 1831. *Reports of Medical Cases.* Vol. 2, *Diseases of the Brain and Central Nervous System.* London: Longman.

Brouwer, Barends. 1920. "The Significance of Phylogenetic and Ontogentic Studies for the Neuropathologist." *Journal of Nervous and Mental Disease* 51:113–23.

Bullock, W. E. 1913. "The Experimental Transmission of Disseminated Sclerosis into Rabbits." *Lancet* 1:1183–85.

Butler, Alban. 1904. *The Lives of the Fathers, Martyrs....* 12 vols. New York: J. Kennedy.

Butler, W. M. 1890. "Disseminated Sclerosis, with Case." *Hahnemannian Monthly* 25:147–51.

Campbell, A. M. G. 1963. "Veterinary Workers and Disseminated Sclerosis." *Journal of Neurology, Neurosurgery and Psychiatry* 26:514–15.

_____, P. Daniel, and R. J. Porter et al. 1947. "Disease of the Nervous System Occurring Among Research Workers on Swayback in Lambs." *Brain* 70:50–58.

Carnegie, P. R., and C. E. Lumsden. 1966. "Encephalitogenic Peptides from Spinal Cord." *Nature* 209:1354.

Carswell, Robert. 1835–38. *Pathological Anatomy: Illustrations of the Elementary Forms of Disease.* (In fascicles.) London: Longman, Orme, Brown, Green and Longman.

Cartwright, Frederick F. 1972. *Disease and History: The Influence of Disease in Shaping the Events of History.* New York: Thomas Y. Crowell.

Chevassut, Kathleen. 1930. "The Etiology of Disseminated Sclerosis." *Lancet* 1:552 59.

Clendenning, Logan. 1942. *Source Book of Medical History.* New York: Dover.

Clymer, Meredith. 1870. "Notes on the Physiology and Pathology of the Central Nervous System." *New York Medical Journal* 11, 3:225–61 and 11, 4.

Cogan, D. G., and S. H. Wray. 1970. "Internuclear Ophthalmoplegia as an Early Sign of Brainstem Tumors." *Neurology* 20:629–33.

Compston, Alastair. 1988. "The 150th Anniversary of the First Depiction of the Lesions of Multiple Sclerosis." *Journal of Neurology, Neurosurgery and Psychiatry* 51:1249–52.

Cotrufo, R., G. Salvati, L. Morcaldi, G. G. Giodano, and G. C. Guazzi. 1969. "Che cosa è malattia di Schilder 1912? Contributo biologico allo studio di un processo neuroendocrino particolare." *Acta Neurologica* 24:301–20.

Davidoff, L. M., B. C. Seegal, and D. Seegal. 1932. "The Arthus Phenomenon: Local Anaphylactic Inflammation in the Rabbit Brain." *Journal of Experimental Medicine* 55:163.

Davies, I. J. T. 1972. *The Practical Significance of the Essential Biological Metals.* Springfield, Illinois: Charles C. Thomas. [63–64, MS and copper, the swayback studies, copper def. predisposes to infect with transmitted agent?]

Dawson, J. W. 1916. "The Histology of Multiple Sclerosis." *Transactions of the Royal Society of Edinburgh* 50:517–740.

DeAlmeida, H. 1991. *Romantic Medicine and John Keats.* New York: Oxford University Press.

Dean, Geoffrey. 1949. "Disseminated Sclerosis in South Africa: Its Relationship to Swayback Disease and Suggested Treatment." *British Medical Journal* 1:842–61.

_____. 1967. "Annual Incidence, Prevalence, Mortality of Multiple Sclerosis in White South African Born and in White Immigrants in South Africa." *British Medical Journal* 1:724–38.

_____. 1988. "Epidemiology of Multiple Sclerosis." In *Trends in European Multiple Sclerosis Research*, ed. Christian Confavreux, Gilbert Almaro, and Michel Devic, pp. 9–20. Amsterdam: Excerpta Medica.

_____, E.I. McDougall, and M. Elian. 1985. "Multiple Sclerosis in Research

Workers Studying Swayback in Lambs: An Updated Report." *Journal of Neurology, Neurosurgery and Psychiatry* 48:859–65.

DeBuck, D., and I. Demeer. 1896. "Un Cas de maladie de Charcot." *Belgique médicine, Grand Haarlem* 1:229–36.

Dercum, F. X. 1883. "Multiple Sclerosis, Traumatic Tremor, Railway Spine." *International Clinics* 1, 3:122–28.

Derry, T. K., and Trevor I. Williams. 1973. *A Short History of Technology.* Oxford: Oxford University Press.

Detels, R., J. A. Brody, and A. H. Edgar. 1972. "Multiple Sclerosis Among American, Japanese and Chinese Migrants to California and Washington." *Journal of Chronic Diseases* 25:3–17.

DeWilde, A. G. 1958. "Etude de l'identification d'un squellette de 15ème siècle." *Extraits des comptes rendus de l'association des anatomistes, 45e Réunion, Gent.*

Dick, G., J. J. McAlister, F. McKeown, and A. M. G. Campbell. 1965. "Multiple Sclerosis and Scrapie." *Journal of Neurology, Neurosurgery and Psychiatry* 28:560–62.

Dristine, F. 1994. "Use of Evoked Potentials in the Diagnosis and Figuration of Multiple Sclerosis." *Clinical Neurosciences* 2:196–201.

Ebers, G. C., K. Kukay, D. E. Bulman et al. 1996. "A Full Genome Search in Multiple Sclerosis." *Nature Genetics* 13:472–76.

Ellenberger, Henri. 1970. *The Discovery of the Unconscious: The History and Evolution of Dynamic Psychiatry.* New York: Basic Books.

Ferraro, A. 1937. "Primary Demyelinating Processes of the Central Nervous System." *Archives of Neurology and Psychiatry* 37:100.

_____, and G. A. Jervis. 1940. "Experimental Disseminated Encephalopathy in the Monkey." *Archives of Neurology and Psychiatry* 43:195.

Finger, Stanley. 1994. *The Origins of Neuroscience: A History of Explorations into Brain Function.* Oxford: Oxford University Press.

Firth, Douglas. 1941. "The Case of Augustus d'Esté (1794–1848): The First Account of Disseminated Sclerosis." *Proceedings of the Royal Society of Medicine* 34:381–84.

_____. 1948. *The Case of Augustus d'Este.* Cambridge: Cambridge University Press.

Fischer, B. H., M. Marks, and T. Reich. 1983. "Hyperbaric Oxygen Treatment of Multiple Sclerosis: A Randomized, Placebo-Controlled, Double Blind Study." *New England Journal of Medicine* 308:181–86.

Foucault, Michel. 1994. *The Birth of the Clinic: An Archaeology of Medical Perception.* Trans. John Sheridan-Smith. New York: Vintage.

Freud, Sigmund. 1963. *Early Psychoanalytic Writings.* New York: Collier Books.

Friedhoff, A. J., and T. M. Chase, eds. 1982. *Gilles de la Tourette's Syndrome.* New York: Raven Press.

Friedman, S. M. et al. 1991. "A Potential Role for Microbial Superantigens in the Pathogenesis of Systemic Autoimmune Disease." *Arthritis and Rheumatism* 34:468–78.

Frommann, Carl. 1864. *Unterschungen über die normale und pathologigische Anatomie des Rückenmarkes.* Jena.

Gallego Moyano, C. 1904. "Enfermedad de Charcot." *Semana medicina, Buenos Aires* 11:1313, 1349.

Gay, D., and G. Dick. 1986. "Is Multiple Sclerosis Caused by an Oral Spirochete?" *Lancet* 2:75.

Georgi, F., and P. Hall. 1960. "Studies on Multiple Sclerosis Frequency in Switzerland and East Africa." *Acta Psychiatrica Scandinavica* 35, supplement 147:75–93.

Gieson, Gerard. 1995. *The Private Science of Louis Pasteur.* Princeton: Princeton University Press.

Gill, J. M. 1904. "A Case of Disseminated Sclerosis of Congenital Origin." *Australasian Medical Gazette* 23:458.

Glaser, Gilbert H. 1978. "Epilepsy, Hysteria and 'Possession': A Historical Essay." *Journal of Nervous and Mental Disease* 166:269.

Goetz, Christopher. 1987. *Charcot, the Clinician: The Tuesday Lessons.* New York: Raven Press.

_____, Michelle Bonduelle and Toby Gelfand. 1995. *Charcot: Constructing Neurology.* New York: Oxford University Press.

Goldberg, B. 1946. "Two Cases of Disseminated Sclerosis in Native Africans." *East African Medical Journal* 33:209–23.

Gonzalez, Juan de Jesus. 1902. "Un caso de escelerosis combinadas." *Cronica médica M Mexicana* 5:58–60.

Good, P. B. 1981. "Has Diabetes Mellitus Ever 'Cured' Multiple Sclerosis?" Brief communication. *Multiple Sclerosis Studies.*

_____. 1988. "MS: A Vascular, Compressive, Metabolic, Toxic and Psychosomatic Bibliography." *Multiple Sclerosis Studies: A Journal of Alternative Hypotheses, Research and Treatments* 1, 1.

Gowers, William. 1868. *A Manual of Diseases of the Nervous System.* London: J. and A. Churchill.

Gray, Landon Carter. 1889. "A Case of Lepto-Meningitis Cerebri Presenting Typical Symptoms of Disseminated Sclerosis." *Journal of Nervous and Mental Disease* 16:92–98.

Gunn, M. 1897. "Discussion of Retro-Ocular Neuritis." *Transactions of the Ophthalmological Society of the United Kingdom* 17:107–217.

_____. 1904. "Retro-Ocular Neuritis." *Lancet* 2:412–13.

Gye, W. E. 1925. "The Etiology of Malignant New Growths." *Lancet* 2:109–16.

Gyldensted, Carsten. 1976. "Computer Tomography of the Brain in Multiple Sclerosis." *Acta Neurologica Scandinavica* 53:386–89.

Hahn, Robert. 1995. *Sickness and Healing: An Anthropological Perspective.* New Haven: Yale University Press.

Hammond, William. 1871a. "Diffused Cerebral Sclerosis." *New York Medical Journal* 13, 2:129–44.

_____. 1871b. "Multiple Cerebral Sclerosis." *American Practitioner* 3:129–50.

Hassin, George. 1942. "The Rise of Neuropathology." *Journal of Neuropathology and Experimental Neurology* 1:1–3.

Heckl, R. W. 1974. "Das Phänomen des inkonstanten Visus bei Multipler Sklerose. Literaturübersicht und Fallstudie mit experimentellen Untersuchungen." *Nervenartz* 45:467–79.

Heine, Heinrich. 1948. *The Poetry and Prose of Heinrich Heine.* Ed. Frederick Ewen. New York: Citadel Press.

Hirschfelder, Joseph. 1882. "Disseminated Sclerosis." *Pacific Medical and Surgical Journal* 25, 10:446–47.

Hoefer, P. F. A., T. J. Putnam, and M. G. Gray. 1938. "Experimental 'Encephalitis' Produced by Intravenous Injection of Various Coagulants." *Archives of Neurology and Psychiatry* 39:799–811.

Huizinga, Jan. 1989. *The Waning of the Middle Ages.* New York: Anchor Doubleday.

Hunt, J. R. 1903. "Multiple Sclerosis with Dementia: A Contribution to the Combination Form of Multiple Sclerosis and Dementia Paralytica." *American Journal of Medical Sciences* 127:974–85.

Hyllestedt, Kay and Leonard T. Kurland, eds. *Further Explorations on the Geographic Distribution of Multiple Sclerosis (Acta Neurologica Scandinavica,* supp. 19, vol. 42, World Federation of Neurologists, Committee on Geographic Neurology, Report of Third Conference). Copenhagen: Munksgaard.

Ingalls, T. H. 1986. "Endemic Clustering of Multiple Sclerosis in Time and Place, 1934–84: Confirmation of Hypothesis." *American Journal of Forensic Medical Pathology* 7:3–21.

Innes, J. R. M. 1939. "Swayback, a Demyelinating Disease of Lambs with Affinities to Schilder's Encephalitis and Its Prevention by Copper." *Journal of Neurology and Psychiatry* 2:323–34.

Irvine, D. G., H. B. Schiefer, and W. J. Hader. 1989. "Geotoxicology of Multiple Sclerosis: The Henribrough, Saskatchewan, Cluster Focus; I, The Water." *Science of the Total Environment* 84:45–59.

Jacob, Alfons. 1921. "Über eine der multiplen Sklerose klinisch nahstehende Erkrankung des Zentralnervensystems (spastische Pseudosklerose) mit bemerkenswerten anatomischen Befunde: Mitteilung eines vierten Falles." *Medizinische Klinik* 17:372.

James, P. B. 1982. "Evidence for Subacute Fat Embolism as the Cause of Multiple Sclerosis." *Lancet* 1:380–86.

Jelinek, J. E. 1994. "Parkinson and the Plum Tree." *Archives of Neurology* 51:1182–83.

Jelliffe, Smith Ely and William Alanson White. 1935. *Diseases of the Central Nervous System.* Philadelphia: Lea and Fletcher.

Jellinek, E. H. 1990. "Heine's Illness: The Case for Multiple Sclerosis." *Journal of the Royal Society of Medicine* 83:516–19.

_____. 1994. "Trauma and Multiple Sclerosis." *Lancet* 343, 895:1053+.

Jervis, G. A. 1943. "Forssman's 'Carotid Syndrome.'" *Archives of Pathology* 35: 560.

_____, A. Ferraro, L. M. Kopeloff and N. Kopeloff. 1941. "Neuropathologic Changes Associated with Experimental Anaphylaxis in Monkeys." *Archives of Neurology and Psychiatry* 45:733.

Johnson, Hillary. 1996. *Osler's Web: Inside the Epidemic of Chronic Fatigue Syndrome.* New York: Basic Books.

Johnson, Keith A., and J. Alex Becker. 1995. *Whole Brain Atlas.* Web page. <http://www.med.harvard.edu>.

Jonez, Hinton. 1951. "Psychotherapy in Multiple Sclerosis (part IV)." *Annals of Allergy* 9:653–57.

_____. 1953. "Allergic Aspects of Multiple Sclerosis." *California Medicine* 79, 5:76–81.

_____, with Miriam Zeller Gross. 1952. *My Fight to Conquer Multiple Sclerosis.* New York: Julian Messmer.

Kabat, E. A., A. Wolf and A. E. Bezer. 1946. "Rapid Production of Acute Disseminated Encephalomyelitis in Rhesus Monkeys by Injection of Brain Tissue with Adjuvants." *Science* 104:362–64.

Kadish, U., and N. Gadoth. 1995. [Heinrich Heine: Death of a poet.] *Harefuah* 128, 6.

Kaplan, Yuri F. 1903. "Sluchai mnozhestvennavo skleroza s preobladynshtshim porazhenivem psikhiki, ili, bit mozhet, pseudoskleroza Westphal'ya." *Russkii Vrach* 2:1212–15.

Keppel Hesselink, J. M. 1991a. "Een monografie van K. F. H. Marx uit 1838: Mogelijk de eerste klinisch-pathologische beschrijving van multipele sclerose." *Nederlands Tijdschrift voor Geneeskund* 135, 51:2439–43.

_____. 1991b. "Een veranderlijk ziektebeeld? De ziekte van Parkinson vanaf 1817." *Nederlands Tijdschrift voor geneeskund* 135, 22:998–1003.

Kesselring, Jürg, ed. 1997. *Multiple Sclerosis.* Cambridge: Cambridge University Press.

Kevles, Bettyann Holtzmann. 1996. *Naked to the Bone: Medical Imaging in the Twentieth Century.* New Brunswick, NJ: Rutgers University Press. (170–71, Kenneth Swanson, discharged Army, diagnosed schiz. or MS, CT scan revealed tumor, 1983 decision CT to be part of standard of care; "until MRI the confusing symptoms of MS could only be verified by autopsy" 194)

Klaniczay, Gabor. 1990. *The Uses of Supernatural Power.* Princeton: Princeton University Press.

Klawans, Harold. 1989. *Toscanini's Fumble and Other Tales of Clinical Neurology.* New York: Bantam.

Klingman, Theophil. 1899. "Histogenesis of Multiple Sclerosis." *Archives of Neurology and Psychiatry* 4:39–64, 193–218.

Kopeloff, N., L. M. Davidoff and L. Kopeloff. 1936. "General and Cerebral Anaphylaxis in the Monkey (Macacus Rhesus)." *Journal of Immunology* 30:16.

[Kozorovitsky, Leonid.] 1992. "How Does the Earth's Magnetic Field Correlate with Multiple Sclerosis?" *Moscow News* 46, 3553 (Nov. 15, 1992): 9. [Theory of physicist Leonid Kozorovitsky: electromagnetic irradiation inhibits muscles' ability to intercept spinal cerebral messages; northern hemisphere solar wind causes magnetosphere disturbances, therefore MS; southern hemisphere free magnetism only over oceans.]

Kurland, Leonard. 1994. "The Evolution of Multiple Sclerosis Epidemiology." *Annals of Neurology* 36, supplement, S2–5.

Kurtzke, John. 1983. "Epidemiology of Multiple Sclerosis." In *Multiple Sclerosis: Pathology, Diagnosis and Management.* Ed. J. F. Hallpike, C. W. M. Adams and W. W. Toutellotte, pp. 47–95. Baltimore: Williams and Wilkins.

Kurtzke, J. F., G. Dean, and D. P. J. Botha. 1970. "A Method for Estimating the Age at Immigration of White Immigrants to South Africa, with an Example of Its Importance." *South African Medical Journal* 44:663–69.

_____, and K. Hyllested. 1975. "Multiple Sclerosis: An Epidemic in the Faroes." *Transactions of the American Neurological Association* 100: 213–15.

Lauer, K. 1995. "Environmental Associations with the Risk of Multiple Sclerosis: The Contribution of Ecological Studies." *Acta Neurologica Scandinavica* Supplement 161:77–88.

Leibowitz, Uri, and Milton Alter. 1969. *Multiple Sclerosis: Keys to Its Cause.* Amsterdam: North Holland Publishing Company.

_____, E. Kahana, and M. Alter. 1969. "Multiple Sclerosis in Immigrant and Native Populations in Israel." *Lancet* 2:1323–34.

Lewis, W. Bevan. 1878. "A Case of Disseminated Cerebral Sclerosis." *Journal of Mental Science* 23:564–65.

Leyden, E. 1893. "J.-M. Charcot." *Deutsche Medizinische Wochenschrift* 45: 151–54.

Lockett, S., and I. A. Nazroo. 1952. "Eye Changes Following Exposure to Metallic Mercury." *Lancet* 1:528–35.

Lumsden, C. E. 1958. "Demyelinating Disease: The Present Situation." *Proceedings of the Royal Society of Medicine* 51:752–55.

McAlpine, Douglas, Charles E. Lumsden, and E. D. Acheson. 1972. *Multiple Sclerosis: A Reappraisal.* Edinburgh and London: Churchill-Livingstone.

McDonald, W. I. 1993. "Multiple Sclerosis." In *The Cambridge World History of Human Disease.* Ed. Kenneth F. Kiple, pp. 883–87. Cambridge: Cambridge University Press.

Mackintosh, A. W. 1903. "A Study of the Modes of Onset in Eighty Cases of Disseminated Sclerosis." *Review of Neurology and Psychiatry (Edinburgh)* 1:73–83.

MacLean, A. R., J. Berkson, H.W. Woltman, and L. Schionneman. 1950. "Multiple Sclerosis in a Rural Community." In *Multiple Sclerosis and the Demyelinating Diseases*, vol. 38, 25–27. Ed. H. W. Woltman. Baltimore: Williams and Wilkins.

Marburg, O. 1905. "Die sogennante akute multiple Sklerose." *Mitteilungen des Gesellschafts für inneren Medizin und Kinderheilkunde* 4:200–201.

Marshall, V. 1988. "Multiple Sclerosis Is a Chronic Central Nervous System Infection Caused by a Spirochetal Agent." *Medical Hypotheses* 25:89–93.

Martin, Russell. 1986. *Matters Gray and White: A Neurologist, His Patients, and the Mysteries of the Brain.* New York: Henry Holt.

Massalongo, Roberto. 1903. "Sclerosi a placche famigliare." *Lavori della Congressa di medicina internale* 13:406–11.

Medaer, R. 1979. "Does the History of Multiple Sclerosis Go Back as Far as the 14th Century?" *Acta Neurologica Scandinavica* 60:189–92.

Meirowitz, P. 1900. "A Case of Atypical Cerebro-Spinal Multiple Sclerosis, Simulating the Combination of Tabes and Progressive Muscular Atrophy." *Post-Graduate Medical Review* 15:668–74.

Merzbacher, Ludwig. 1904. "Weitere Mitteilungen über eine eigenartige hereditäre familiäre Erkrankung des Zentralnervensystems." *Medizinische Klinik* 4:1952–55.

Mettler, Cecilia. 1947. *History of Medicine.* Philadelphia: Blakiston Company.

Mettler, L. H. 1905. "Case of Disseminated Cerebrospinal Sclerosis, with a Suggestive Family History." *Chicago Medical Recorder* 27:290–93.

Micale, Mark. 1993. "On the 'Disappearance' of Hysteria: A Study in the Clinical Deconstruction of a Diagnosis." *Isis* 84:496–526.

Moxon, Walter. 1875a. "Eight Cases of Insular Sclerosis of the Brain and Spinal Cord." *Guy's Hospital Reports*, series 3, 20:437–78.

_____. 1875b. "Two Cases of Insular Sclerosis of the Brain and Spinal Cord." *Lancet* 3:471–72.

Müller, R. 1949. "Studies on Disseminated Sclerosis." *Acta Medica Scandinavica* 133, supplement, 1–214.

Nanji, A. A., and S. Narod. 1986. "Multiple Sclerosis, Latitude and Dietary Fat: Is Pork the Missing Link?" *Medical Hypotheses* 20:279–88.

Neff, Irwin H., and Theophil Klingmann. 1899. "A Case of Multiple Cerebro-Spinal Sclerosis of a Special Anatomical Form, with a History of Pronounced Family Defect." *American Journal of Insanity* 56:431–45.

Nettleship, E. 1884. "On Cases of Retro-Ocular Neuritis." *Transactions of the Ophthalmological Society of the United Kingdom* 4:186–226.

Nicolson, Malcolm, and Cathleen McLaughlin. 1988. "Social Construction-ism and Medical Sociology: A Study of the Vascular Theory of Multiple Sclerosis." *Sociology of Health and Illness* 10, 3:234–61.

Noyes, Henry D. 1871. "A Case of Supposed Disseminated Sclerosis of the Brain and Spinal Cord." *Archives of Scientific and Practical Medicine* 1, 1:43–46.

Ollivier d'Angers, C. P. 1824. *De la moelle épinière et de ses maladies.* Paris: Crevot.

Oppenheim, H. 1896. "Zur Lehre von multiplen Sklerose." *Berline Klinische Wochenschrift* 33:184–89.

Palmer, F. S. 1904. "The Early Manifestations of Insular Sclerosis, with a Table Showing the Modes of Onset in Fifty Cases." *Medical Press and Circular,* new series, 78:243–47.

Parinaud, Henri. 1884. "Troubles oculaires de la sclérose en plaques." *Journal de Santé* 3:3–5.

Pawel, Ernst. 1995. *The Poet Dying: Heinrich Heine's Last Years in Paris.* New York: Farrar, Straus and Giroux.

Pelizaeus, Friedrich. 1885. "Über eine eigentümliche Form spasticher Läh-mung mit cerebraler scheinnungen auf hereditärer Grundlage (multiple sklerose)." *Archiv Psychiatrie und Nervenkrankheit* 16:698–710.

Perkin, G. P., and F. Clifford Rose. 1979. *Optic Neuritis and Its Differential Diagnosis.* Oxford: Oxford University Press.

Plummer, William. 1995. "The Enemy Within: Once Fierce Rivals, Three Olympic Skiers Now Fight a Common Foe — Multiple Sclerosis." *People Weekly,* November 13, pp. 153+ (Jimmie Heuga, Egon Zimmerman, Josef "Pepi" Stiegler —1964 Olympic skiers, Innsbruck).

Pohlen, K. 1942. [Summary.] *Statistical Bulletin* 2, 4 & 5.

Poser, C. M. 1994. "The Dissemination of Multiple Sclerosis, a Viking Saga: A Historical Essay." *Annals of Neurology,* 36, supplement 2:231–43.

_____. 1995. "Viking Voyages: The Origin of Multiple Sclerosis? An Essay in Medical History." *Acta Neurologica Scandinavica,* supplement 161:11–22.

_____. 1996. "Multiple Sclerosis." In Shakir, Newman, and Poser 1996:537–55.

_____, and L. Van Bogaert. 1956. "The Natural History and Evolution of the Concept of Schilder's Diffuse Sclerosis." *Acta Scandinavica Psychiatrica et Neurologica* 31:285.

Poskanzer, D. C., J. L. Sheridan, L. B. Prenney, and A. M. Walker. 1980. "Multiple Sclerosis in the Orkney and Shetland Islands: II, The Search for an Exogenous Etiology." *Journal of Epidemiology and Community Health* 34:240–52.

Putnam, J. J. 1897. "A Group of Cases of Scleroses of the Spinal Cord, Asso-ciated with Diffuse Collateral Degeneration, Occuring with Enfeebled Persons Past Middle Life, and Especially in Women; Studied with Par-ticular Reference to Etiology." *Journal of Nervous and Mental Disease,* new series 16: 69–110.

Putnam, T. J. 1937. "Evidences of Vascular Occlusion in Multiple Sclerosis and 'Encephalomyelitis.'" *Archives for Neurology and Psychiatry* 27:1298–1307.

_____, et al. 1947. *Multiple Sclerosis, Diagnosis and Treatment: Manual of Information for Use of Physicians Only.* New York: National Multiple Sclerosis Society.

_____, Ludwig V. Chiavacci, Hans Hoff, and Hyman G. Weitzen. 1947. "Results of Treatment of Multiple Sclerosis with Dicoumarin." *Archives of Neurology and Psychiatry* 57:3–11.

_____, J. B. McKenna, and J. Evans. 1932. "Experimental Multiple Sclerosis in Dogs from Injections of Tetanus Toxin." *Journal for Psychiatry and Neurology* 44:460–71.

_____, J. B. McKenna, and L. R. Morrison. 1931. "Studies in Multiple sclerosis: I, The Histogenesis of Experimental Multiple Sclerosis Plaques and Their Relation to Multiple Sclerosis." *Journal of the American Medical Association* 97:1591–96.

Réthi, L. 1907. *Die Laryngrealen Erscheinungen bei Multipler Sklerose des Gehirns und Rückenmarks.* Vienna: Josef Šafář.

Reynolds, Ernest S. 1904. "Some Cases of Family Disseminated Sclerosis." *Brain* 27:163–69.

Rhodes, Richard. 1997. *Deadly Feasts: Tracking the Secrets of a Terrifying New Plague.* New York: Simon and Schuster.

Rindfleisch, E. 1863. "Histologisches detail in der grauen degeneration von Gehirn und Rückenmark." *Virchows Archiv* 26:474–83.

Rivers, T. M, D. H. Sprunt, and G. P. Berry. 1935. "Observations on Attempts to Produce Acute Disseminated Encephalomyelitis in Monkeys." *Journal of Experimental Medicine* 58:39–45.

_____, and Francis F. Schwentker. 1935. "Encephalomyelitis Accompanied by Myelin Destruction Experimentally Produced in Monkeys." *Journal of Experimental Medicine* 61:689–702.

Robin, Charles. 1864. *Programme du cours de histologie.*

Rodriguez-Arias, B. 1953. "Insulin Therapy in Multiple Sclerosis." *Journal of the American Medical Association* 152:1486–89.

Rohowsky-Kochan, Christine. 1995. "Canine Distemper Virus-Specific Antibodies in MS." *Neurology* 45, 9:1554–69.

Rose, F. Clifford, and W. F. Bynum, eds. 1982. *Historical Aspects of the Neurosciences.* New York: Raven Press.

Russell, J. S. Risien. 1899. "Disseminate Sclerosis." In *Allbutt's System of Medicine,* vol. 7, pp. 50–96. London

Sachs, Bernard, and E. D. Friedman. 1922. "General Symptomatology and Differential Diagnosis of Multiple Sclerosis." *Archives of Neurology and Psychiatry* 7, 5:551–60.

Sanz, Cynthia. 1995. "The Challenge of His Life (Joe Hartzler, lead prosecutor in the Oklahoma City bombing case and a victim of MS)." *People Weekly* October 16: pp. 169+.

Schaltenberg, G. 1938. "Neurere anschauungen über die ureachen und behandlung der Multiplen Sklerose." *Medizinische Welt* 12:435–43.

Scherb, Georges. 1904. "Syndrome cérébelleux de Babinski ou sclérose en plaques?" *Bulletin médicale de l'Algérie* 15:74–77. Reprinted with revisions.

_____. 1905a. "Sclérose en plaques frustes ou syndrome cérébelleux de Babinski?" *Nouvelle Iconographie de la Salpêtrière* 18:31–35 (with photo).

_____. 1905b. "Sclérose en plaques simulant la maladie de Charcot." *Bulletin médicale de l'Algérie* 16:56–58, abstracted in *Revue neurologique 1904*, 12:1152.

Schilder, Paul. 1912. "Zur Kenntnis der sogennanten Diffusensklerosen." *Zeitschrift Gesamte von Neurologie und Psychiatrie* 10:1–5.

Schüle, Wilhelm. 1870. "Beitrag zur Multiplen Sklerose des Gehirns und Rückenmarks." *Deutsches Archiv für klinischer Medizin* 7:259.

Seguin, E. C. 1878. "A Contribution to the Pathological Anatomy of Disseminated Cerebro-Spinal Sclerosis." *Journal of Nervous and Mental Disease*, new series, 5:281–93.

Selhorst, J. B., and R. F. Saul. 1995. "Uhthoff and His Syndrome." *Journal of Neuro-ophthalmology* 15, 2:63–69.

Shakir, Raad A., Peter K. Newman, and Charles M. Poser, eds. 1996. *Tropical Neurology*. London: W.B. Saunders.

Shorter, Edward. 1992. *From Paralysis to Fatigue: A History of Psychosomatic Illness in the Modern Era*. New York: Free Press.

Sinkler, William. 1902. "A Case Exhibiting the Symptoms of Both Tabes and Multiple Sclerosis." *Philadelphia Medical Journal* 10:599.

Smith, Dian G. 1995. "Respect for the Dead." *Journal of the American Medical Association* 274 (November): 1408.

Smith, Elisabeth. 1995. *Illness Narrative Among Multiple Sclerosis Patients: The Social, Cultural and Semiotic Phenomena of Diagnosis, Adaptation and the Doctor-Patient Relationship*. Senior honors thesis, Dartmouth College, Hanover, N.H.

Spillane, John D., ed. 1973. *Tropical Neurology*. Oxford: Oxford University Press.

_____. 1981. *The Doctrine of the Nerves: Chapters in the History of Neurology*. Oxford: Oxford University Press.

Stein, E. C., R. B. Schiffer, W. J. Hall, and N. Young. 1987. "Multiple Sclerosis and the Workplace: Report of an Industry-Based Cluster." *Neurology* 37:1672.

Steiner, Gabriel. 1962. *Multiple Sklerose: Ihre Aetiologie, Pathologie, Pathogenose und Therapie*. Berlin: Springer Verlag.

Stenager, Egon. 1992. "Schilder's or Stohr's Disease." *Journal of the History of the Neurosciences* 1:163–66.

_____. 1996. "The Course of Heine's Illness: Diagnostic Considerations." *Journal of Medical Biography* 4, 1:28–32.

Strümpell, Albrecht. 1898. "Über die Westphal'sche Pseudoskleröse und über diffuse Hirnsklerose, inbesondere bei Kindern." *Deutsche Zeitschrift für Nervenheilkunden* 12:115–49.

_____. 1900. "Historische Notiz betreffend die Pseudosklerose." *Deutsche Zeitschrift für Nervenheilkunde* 16:497.

Surgeon General's Office, United States Army. 1906. *Index-Catalogue of the Library of the Surgeon-General's Office, United States Army, second series.* Washington, D.C.: Government Printing Office.

Symonds, C. P. 1975. "Multiple Sclerosis and the Swayback Story." *Lancet* 1:155–56.

Talley, Colin Lee. 1995. "A Most Mysterious Disease: A Cultural History of Multiple Sclerosis, 1868–1958." Master's thesis, University of California–San Francisco.

Taylor, E. W. 1922. "Multiple Sclerosis: The Localization of Lesions with Respect to Symptoms." *Archives of Neurology and Psychiatry* 7:561–83.

Teague, Oscar. 1922. "Bacteriological Investigation of Multiple Sclerosis." In *Multiple Sclerosis*, ed. Association for Research in Nervous and Mental Diseases. New York: Paul B. Hoeber.

Temple, Donald. 1994. *Brain Analysis and the French Connection, 1791–1841.* New York: Raven Press.

Tienari, P., L. Peltonen, and J. Palo. 1993. "Genetic Susceptibility to MS Linked to Myelin Basic Protein." *Lancet* 2:256.

Turner, P. 1986. "A Small-Town Disease." *Science* 86, 7:72–73.

Uhthoff, W. 1890. "Unterschungen über die bei der Multiplen Herdsklerose vorkommenden Augenstorungen." *Archiv der Psychiatrie und Nervenkrankheit* 21:55–116, 303–410.

Utz, U., et al. 1993. "Skewed T-Cell Receptor in Genetically Identical Twins Correlates with Multiple Sclerosis." *Nature* 364:243–47.

Valentiner, T. 1856. "Über die Sclerose des Gehirns und Rückenmarks." *Deutsche Klinik* 14.

Van Wart, Robert M. 1905. "A Note of the Frequency of Multiple Sclerosis in Louisiana." *New Orleans Medical and Surgical Journal* 57:549–51.

Virchow, Rudolf. (1858) 1971. *Cellular Pathology, as Based on Physical and Pathological Evidence.* Trans. Frank Chance. New York: Dover.

Waksman, B. H. 1995. "More Genes Versus Environment." *Nature* 377:105–6.

Warren, H. V. 1974. "Environmental Lead: A Survey of Its Possible Physiological Significance." *Journal of Biosocial Sciences* 6:223–47.

Warren, S. A., and K. G. Warren. 1982. "Multiple Sclerosis and Diabetes Mellitus: Further Evidence of a Relationship." *Canadian Journal of Neurological Sciences* 9:415–20.

Weil, Arthur. 1931. "A Study of the Etiology of Multiple Sclerosis." *Journal of the American Medical Association* 97, 22:1587–91.

Wellingham-Jones, Patricia. 1991. "Characteristics of Handwriting of Subjects with Multiple Sclerosis." *Perceptual and Motor Skills* 73, 3 (December): 867.

Westphal, Carl. 1888. "Über Multiple Sclerosen bei zwei Knaben." *Charité-Annalen* 13:459–70.

Winfield, J. B., and W. N. Jarfour. 1991. "Stress Proteins, Autoimmunity and Autoimmune Disease." *Current Topics in Microbiology and Immunology* 167:161–89.

Winkelman, N. W., and N. Gotten. 1935. "Encephalomyelitis Following the Use of Serum and Vaccine." *American Journal of Syphilis and Neurology* 19:414.

Wisniewski, H. M. 1972. "Patterns of Myelin Damage Resulting from Inflammatory and Toxin-Induced Lesions and Their Relationship to Multiple Sclerosis." In *Multiple Sclerosis: Immunology, Virology and Ultrastructure*, F. Wolfgram, G.W. Ellison, J.G. Stevens, and J.M. Andrews, ed. New York: Academic Press.

Wojtowicz, S. 1993. "Multiple Sclerosis and Prions." *Medical Hypotheses* 40:48–54.

Wolf, A., E. A. Kabat, and A. E. Bezer. 1946. "The Pathology of Acute Disseminated Encephalomyelitis Produced Experimentally in the Rhesus Monkey and Its Resemblance to Human Demyelinating Disease." *Journal of Neuropathology and Experimental Neurology* 6:333–41.

Wolfgram, Frederick. 1979. "What If Multiple Sclerosis Isn't an Immunological or a Viral Disease? The Case for a Circulating Toxin." *Neurochemical Research* 4:1–14.

Wood, H. C. 1878. "The Multiple Scleroses." *Medical Recorder* 14:224.

Wordsworth, William, ed. 1983. *Jacqueline du Pré: Impressions*. New York: Vanguard.

Wynn, D. R., M. Rodriguez, W. M. O'Fallon, and L. T. Kurland. 1989. "Update on the Epidemiology of Multiple Sclerosis." *Mayo Clinic Proceedings* 64:808–17.

Young, I. R., A. S. Hall, C. A. Pallis et al. 1981. "Nuclear Magnetic Resonance Imaging of the Brain in Multiple Sclerosis." *Lancet* 2:1063–67.

Zhu, Han-ying. 1984. "Multiple Sclerosis." In *Modern Chinese Medicine*, Vol. 2: *Chinese Medicine*, ed. Wu He-guang, pp. 404–7. Lancaster, Pa.: MTP Press.

Zipp, F., F. Weber, S. Huber et al. 1995. "Genetic Control of Multiple Sclerosis: Increased Production of Lymphotoxin and Tumor Necrosis Factor-Alpha by HLA-DR2(+) T Cells." *Annals of Neurology* 38:723–30.

Index